Keto Meal Prep 2021:

The Complete Guide to Keto Meal Prep for Beginners: Burn Fat, Save Money, Save Time, and Live Your Best Life

Tyler MacDonald

Table of Contents

Introduction

Finding time to prepare healthy meals at home can be a pain, right? You work all day long. You may have children to take care of. You could even be trying to take college courses. With life hitting you from everywhere, when are you supposed to have time to cook? Maybe you have the time to cook, but you want to save money and time so that you can do things with your family or hit the gym.

Chances are that you have a lot that you want to accomplish while also getting healthier. A ketogenic diet is a great option for getting healthy, but it can seem overwhelming at first. There are a lot of people who are in your position. The great news is that learning keto meal prepping will solve your problems.

Throughout this book, you learn about the ketogenic diet as well as meal prep. You will learn exactly what it means to be keto, and how you will lose weight, get healthy, and improve your life with the help of this low-carb high-fat. The list of benefits associated with the ketogenic diet is nearly endless.

The main reason people fail when they first start on a ketogenic diet is that they don't have easy access to keto-friendly meals. This is especially true for the busy person. They end up not having enough time to make their meals. When you start using meal prepping, it will make this a hundred times easier. For those who have never heard of or tried meal prepping, a simple explanation is that you make all of your meals in advance. Meal prep is essentially homemade TV dinners.

Meal prepping has gained in popularity, and it is only going to continue to grow. Meal prepping gives you more control over what you consume, and it guarantees you a healthy meal that is just a freezer away. Keto meal prepping aims to help make the ketogenic diet easier so that you won't be so quick to turn to non-keto, processed, and packaged foods. This is extremely simple to execute, and you will quickly see the benefits in as little as a week.

The book has three two-week meal prep plans for the beginner, performance minded, and for maintenance. Besides that, there will be several other recipes to follow the meal prep plans. You will also find nutrition information so that you no longer need to worry about figuring it out on your own.

Thank you for choosing *Keto Meal Prep 2021*. Now, if you are ready to get started and feel amazing, let's continue.

The Ketogenic Diet and Its Benefits

Why is everyone so crazy about the keto diet? Well, this low-carb diet focuses on you consuming lots of healthy fats while lowering your intake of carbs. You get your energy from consuming only 75 percent fats, 20 percent protein, and 5 percent carbs. This means you are only allowed to eat 20 to 50 grams of carbs each day.

This diet was named for the metabolic process called ketosis, where the body changes its fuel source from carbs to fat that has been stored in the body. The goal of this diet is to force the body into ketosis, which causes your liver to begin producing ketones that will run your body. You aren't starving yourself; you are just keeping carbs away from the body. This could cause improved focus, fast weight loss, better physical health, and improved mental clarity.

The ketogenic diet is a bit like the Atkins diet or any other low carb diets. Once you change the body's fuel source, the body's metabolism will change, and this makes you feel more energized.

Benefits

The ketogenic diet does offer many benefits. Here are a few of the big ones:

- *Increased Muscle Mass:* This diet is great if you are looking to increase your muscle mass because you are eating more protein.

- *Anti-Aging:* Your skin and body will feel and look younger when you follow this diet.

- *Decreased Inflammation:* This diet produces ketone bodies. The body burns these ketone bodies better than carbs and, in turn, creates fewer free radicals and less oxidation that damages cell membranes and thus reduces inflammation.

- *Better Skin:* Many people have noticed this diet helps soften their skin and can clear up acne.

- *Increases Energy:* The keto diet improves mitochondrial function by producing fewer free radicals.

- *Improves Brain Function:* Since the brain runs better off ketones, this diet can help with problems focusing and brain fog.

- *Reduces the Risk of Many Diseases:* If you have any of the following conditions, this diet could help improve them:

- High Blood Pressure
- Fatty Liver Disease
- Migraines
- Cancer
- Heart Disease
- Obesity
- Parkinson's Disease
- Chronic Inflammation
- Alzheimer's Disease
- Type 1 Diabetes
- Type 2 Diabetes
- Epilepsy

- *Quick Weight Loss:* When you begin the keto diet, you could lose up to ten pounds in your first week. This loss will mainly be excess water weight. After this quick weight reduction, you could lose up to two pounds per week from there.

Maintaining the Ketogenic Diet

This diet encourages you to eat fresh foods such as healthy oils and fats, vegetables, fish, and meats. You will be reducing all chemically-treated and processed foods. You can do this diet for a long time and even enjoy it. This is essential if you want to lose weight and help with the above conditions. What isn't to love about a diet that lets you eat eggs and bacon for breakfast?

Every study that has been done shows this diet can help people feel fuller longer, have more energy through the day and lose weight. Feeling fuller longer and having more energy comes from the biggest part of your daily calories coming from fats that are digested slower and denser in calories. Because of this, most people who follow this diet will eat fewer calories since they feel fuller longer and don't have cravings.

Why Keto?

Once you begin eating a ketogenic diet, your body will get better at burning fats for fuel. This is wonderful for many reasons. The main reason is that fats have more calories than carbs, which keeps you from eating so much food. Your body easily burns all the fat that has been stored, which is what you want to get rid of. This, in turn, results in losing more weight. Burning fat for fuel gives you constant energy and won't cause spikes in your blood glucose. You won't be experiencing the lows and highs you get when eating huge amounts of carbs. Having constant energy levels during your day means you will get more done and won't feel as tired.

Along with these benefits, following a keto diet can also help with:

- Improve brain function

- Improves good or HDL levels of cholesterol

- Reduces bad or LDL levels of cholesterol

- Reduces blood pressure

- Reduces triglyceride levels

- Reduces insulin resistance and blood sugar

- Results in losing more body fat.

What About Diabetics?

If you have been diagnosed with diabetes, you can still do a low carb diet. It could start reversing the condition for anyone who has type 2 diabetes, and for people who have type 1 diabetes, it could improve the way your body controls blood sugar.

Always talk with your doctor before starting a low carb diet, especially if you have type 1 diabetes. If you take medicines to help control your insulin levels, you might have to decrease your dose. Your physician might suggest you begin this diet under their supervision so they can check your blood glucose levels and change up your dose of insulin if needed. If you have type 1 diabetes, you need to eat over 50 grams of carbs each day to keep you from going into ketoacidosis.

Ketoacidosis is a metabolic state that becomes toxic when your body can't regulate its production of ketones. This causes a large accumulation of keto acids that causes the blood's pH to decrease drastically and makes the blood acidic. The main causes of ketoacidosis are extreme starvation, prolonged alcoholism, and type 1 diabetes. This could result in starvation ketoacidosis, alcoholic ketoacidosis, and diabetic ketoacidosis. Ketoacidosis usually doesn't happen for any reason other than being a type 1 diabetic.

Living with Ratios

The keto diet was built on ratios, just like the Food Pyramid. It is extremely important to consume the correct balance of macronutrients so your body gets the energy that is needed so you aren't missing any essential protein or fat.

Foods are made of macronutrients. These include carbohydrates, protein, and fats. Every macronutrient gives you a specific amount of energy for every gram that is eaten.

- Carbs will give you around four calories per gram.

- Protein gives you around four calories per gram.

- Fats give you about nine calories per gram.

With this diet, the calories you should get from fats need to be about 65 to 75 percent. The calories from protein need to be around 20 to 25 percent, and the last five percent comes from carbs.

The number of calories you consume all depends on a few different factors:

- Do you want to gain muscle?

- Do you want to maintain the muscles you have?

- Do you want to lose weight?

- The types of workout you do: cardio, weight lifting, or both

- The number of hours you do the above each week.

- Your daily activity level: are you a pro athlete, wait tables, sit behind a desk.

- Your current body weight (lean): the body fat subtracted from the total weight.

You can find a calculator online that will give you your daily macro levels. You can find one by doing a quick search for "keto calculator." These will allow you to quickly and easily put in your numbers and get an estimate for your specific caloric needs.

A great thing about this diet is it isn't important to track every number to reach your goal. If you would like to track it that way, it is a good way to increase your progress. By keeping track, you will get a reminder every day to stay on course.

Nutrients that are Needed

You absolutely have to drink a lot of water when you start the keto diet. You might even realize you are going to the bathroom more often, and this is perfectly normal because your body is getting rid of all your water weight.

This occurs since you have cut out many processed foods and have begun consuming more whole foods. Processed foods are loaded with sodium, and when you change up your diet suddenly, it causes a quick drop in your sodium intake.

When you reduce your carb intake, it lowers your insulin levels. This sends a message to your kidneys to get rid of excess sodium. Because the body is getting rid of stored sodium, your body starts getting rid of a lot of water, and your body might become low on electrolytes and sodium.

Once this happens, you might have symptoms like nausea, irritability, runny nose, coughing, headaches, and fatigue. This is commonly called the "keto flu." You must understand this isn't the actual influenza virus. This is called the "keto flu" because of the similar symptoms to the actual flu. It isn't a real virus or contagious.

Most people who experience these symptoms think this diet is what made them sick and start eating carbs again. This "flu phase" means your body is having withdrawals from processed foods, carbs, and sugar. It is learning to use fat as fuel. The "keto flu" only last a couple of days while your body gets adjusted. You can lessen these symptoms by adding more electrolytes and sodium into your diet.

Getting Ready

Now that you have the information behind the science and benefits of the ketogenic diet, you are ready to start. In the remaining chapters, you are going to get all the information you will need to succeed with this diet, including recipes, meal plans, what foods to stay away from, and what foods to buy.

Ketosis and Its Effects

When you eat a high carb diet, your body is in glycolysis, which is a metabolic state. This means that the majority of the energy your body expends comes from the glucose in your blood. When you are in this state, and after you have eaten, your blood glucose spikes and creates high insulin levels. This causes your body to store fat. This, in turn, keeps your body from releasing the fat it has stored in its tissues.

Ketosis is a natural state your body enters when it gets fueled by fat. This can happen when you fast or are following a strict low carb diet.

There are many benefits to being in ketosis, like weight loss, performance, and health. These can come with some side effects. For people who have type 1 diabetes or other diseases, excessive ketosis can become dangerous.

When you are in ketosis, your body will produce ketones. These are small fuel molecules that the body uses as fuel when the body's glucose supplies are short. Your fat reserves will continuously be released and then consumed. Your liver will begin converting fat into ketones that get released into the bloodstream. Your body will use these just like glucose. The brain can be fueled by ketones, too.

Getting into Ketosis

There are two ways for the body to reach ketosis: following a ketogenic diet or fasting. With either of these circumstances, when the body's glucose gets depleted, the body switches its fuel source to fat. Insulin, which is a hormone that stores fat, when it becomes low, and your body is burning fat, its ability to burn fat will increase. This means that your body will have better access to your fat stores and be able to get rid of them.

You can consider yourself in ketosis when your body produces enough ketones to make a significant level in the blood, usually more than .5 millimeters. The fastest way for this to happen is by fasting, but you can't fast forever.

This is why most people begin a ketogenic diet since you can eat this diet for an indefinite amount of time.

The goal of this diet is to keep you in ketosis at all times. If you are just beginning this diet, to get your body into ketosis could take anywhere from one to two months.

When your body has gotten into ketosis, the glucose your body has stored in your liver and muscles will decrease, your energy levels will be higher, your muscle endurance will increase, and you will have less water weight. If you knock yourself out of ketosis due to eating too many carbs, you can return to ketosis faster than before. When your body becomes adapted to the diet, you can increase your carb intake to 50 grams of carbohydrates each day and still stay in ketosis.

Reaching Optimal Levels of Ketosis

This is the point everyone who does this diet wants to reach. Once you have reached optimal ketosis, your body burns fat at the fastest speed it can. In order to get to this level, you have to follow this diet, as stated in this book. There aren't any tricks that will help you reach this level, but there are certain things you can do.

Here are the various levels of ketones you could have:

- Under 0.5 means you aren't in ketosis.

- Between 0.5 and 1.5 is a light level of ketosis. In this range, you will lose weight, but it isn't going to be optimal.

- About 1.5 to 3 is considered optimal and is best for maximum weight loss.

- Levels over 3 are unnecessary. High levels won't help you in any way. It might harm you since it might mean you are not eating enough food.

Many people think that they are following a strict diet but are surprised when they measure their ketone levels. When they measure them, the ketone levels measure about 0.2 or 0.5, which is nowhere near the sweet spot.

The trick to getting over this plateau is you have to steer clear of all the obvious sources of carbs but make sure your intake of protein doesn't go higher than your intake of fats. It has been said that protein won't change your glucose levels as carbs will, but if you eat too many, especially if you consume more protein than fat, it will affect your glucose levels. This is going to compromise your optimal ketosis.

The secret to working around this problem is to increase your fat intake. This can easily be done by adding a large dollop of herbed butter to the top of your steak. This can keep you from eating too much or eating a second helping.

You could also start your day with a cup of keto coffee to help you not feel hungry before lunch and help you not eat as much protein. You'll find the recipe later on in the book.

The more fat you consume, the fuller you are going to feel. This makes sure you don't eat too much protein, and you are going to eat fewer carbs. This will help you reach optimal ketosis.

Ketosis and Ketoacidosis

There are so many misconceptions about ketosis. The biggest one is confusing it with ketoacidosis. This is a dangerous but rare condition that usually only happens to people who have type 1 diabetes. There are some health care professionals that mix these two up. The main reason might be because their names are similar and there isn't a lot of information on the differences between the two.

Ketosis, as stated above, is a normal state that the body can control. Ketoacidosis is where the body malfunctions because it has created an excessive and unregulated amount of ketones. This can cause things such as vomiting, stomach pain, and nausea. This is then followed by confusion and possibly a coma. This requires urgent medical treatment that might even become fatal.

Ketoacidosis occurs when ketones reach a level of 10 millimolar or more. People that follow a keto diet usually only reach a level of three millimolar or less. Many people struggle to reach 0.5. Long-term fasting, which means you haven't consumed food for over one week, could bring that number up to six.

If you have a pancreas that functions properly and produces insulin correctly, you don't have type 1 diabetes. It is going to be extremely hard for you to reach ketoacidosis even if you tried. This won't happen because your body releases insulin when your body produces too many ketones, which shuts down ketone production. Since type 1 diabetes prevents insulin production, their bodies can't regulate overactive ketones.

Brain Fuel

Many people think you need to eat carbs to have fuel for your brain. Our brains will happily burn carbs when you eat them, but when carbs become unavailable, it will happily eat ketones.

This is needed for basic survival because our bodies can only store carbs for a couple of days. The brain might shut down after a few days without food. Alternatively, it needs to convert muscle protein quickly into glucose, which isn't efficient just to keep working. This means we might waste away very fast. If this was how our bodies worked, humans would not have survived before food became available 24 hours a day and seven days a week.

Our bodies have evolved to work a lot smarter than that. Normally, our bodies will store fat that will last so we can survive several weeks without any food. Ketosis is what happens to make sure our brains can run on these fat stores.

Measuring Ketosis

When you begin the keto diet, you need to know when you are in ketosis. This will create a big boost in your confidence. Testing lets you know whether or not you are following the diet correctly.

There are a few ways to help you figure out whether or not you have reached ketosis. The first way to measure ketones is by testing your blood. This means you have to buy a meter and requires you to prick your finger.

There are a few reasonably priced gadgets out there that can help you with this, and it only takes a few seconds to figure out what your blood ketone level is. Many people won't go to this extreme, but it is the most accurate and effective.

You need to measure your blood ketones first thing every morning on a fasted stomach. You can compare them with the levels that were listed earlier in this chapter to see if you are or aren't in ketosis.

These meters will measure the amount of BHB you have in your blood. This is the main ketone that is present in the blood when you are in ketosis. The downside of this method is having to prick your finger to get blood.

Finding a kit will cost about $30 to $40, with another $5 for each test strip. This is why most people who choose this test only perform a test weekly or every other week.

If your budget doesn't allow you to purchase a blood ketone meter, there are other options that will help you figure out whether or not you have reached ketosis.

1. Insomnia

A huge issue for many keto followers is having insomnia, especially when they are just beginning this diet. When a person reduces their carb intake drastically, it could cause sleeping problems. As with everything else, this too shall pass.

2. Short-term fatigue

When your body is making the initial switch into ketosis, it could cause weakness and fatigue, making it hard for many people to stick with it. This is a normal side effect but one that lets you know you are reaching ketosis.

This crappy feeling might last for one week up to one month before you reach full ketosis. In order to reduce this feeling, you could take an electrolyte supplement or add more salt to your diet.

3. Digestive issues

Because of all the changes in the foods you are eating, you may experience some constipation or diarrhea when just starting. This lets you know that you are reaching ketosis. Once this transition period is over, these issues should go away.

4. *Short-term performance decrease*

Just like number two above, fatigue could cause a decrease in your exercise performance. This is because of the reduction in the glycogen stores in your muscles that gave you the fuel you needed to do high-intensity exercises. After a week or two, your performance levels should return to normal.

5. *Appetite suppression*

Many people report that their hunger decreases when they follow a ketogenic diet. The reason behind this is still being researched. It is believed that this reduction in hunger is caused by the increase in protein and vegetable consumption, along with the changes in your hunger hormones. These ketones might affect the way your brain reacts to hunger.

6. *Better focus and energy*

Many people sometimes report feeling tired, sick, or having brain fog when they begin a keto diet. This is called the keto flu, but people who follow this for a long time report increased focus and better energy. Your body needs time to adapt to any new diet. When you hit ketosis, your brain begins burning ketones for energy, and this might take a week or two for it to begin happening.

Ketones are a powerful fuel source for the brain as opposed to carbs. This means it will improve your mental clarity and brain function.

7. *Ketones in your breath and urine*

If you don't like the thought of pricking your finger, you can measure blood ketones by using a breath analyzer. This monitors for acetone, one of the three ketones present in the blood when you have reached ketosis. The other two are beta-hydroxybutyrate and acetoacetate.

This lets you know when your ketone levels are in ketosis since acetone only leaves your body when you reach ketosis. Breath analyzers are fairly accurate but not as accurate as a blood monitor.

Another way to check for ketosis is by checking for ketones in your urine daily using special strips. These are cheap and quick to use to see where your ketone levels are each day. These aren't very reliable.

8. *Bad breath*

This doesn't sound appealing, but many people have said they have bad breath when they hit ketosis. This is a normal side effect. Some people have said that their breath tastes fruitier.

The reason behind this is the elevated ketone levels. The main culprit is acetone that our bodies will excrete through our breath and urine. You might not like the thoughts of having bad breath, but it's a great way to know you are in ketosis.

Many people will brush their teeth many times throughout the day or chew sugar-free gum.

9. Weight loss

This is the most obvious way to know that you are in ketosis. When you are just beginning a keto diet, you are going to have a quick drop in weight, but this is normally water weight. Once you have another drop in weight, this will be your fat stores being used. This is another way you know you are in ketosis.

There are many different signs and symptoms that help you know when you are in ketosis and following the diet correctly. Basically, if you follow the rules for a keto diet and you stay consistent, your body will be in some form of ketosis.

If you want to know for certain whether or not you are in ketosis, the best way to do this is by using a blood ketone monitor.

If you follow this diet for a long time, you don't have to constantly check your ketone levels. After a few weeks, you will know if you are eating right, and it will be easy to remain in ketosis.

Keto Kitchen Staples

Now that you know the science behind this diet and the reasons it works, you are going to learn how to start it and maximize your success. Here is an easy guide for you to use when starting this diet. You can even look back at this any time in your journey for guidance and support.

Clean out the Pantry

You've heard the old saying: "Out with the old, in with the new." Keeping unhealthy, tempting foods inside your house is the largest factor of failing when you begin any diet. If you want to succeed, you have to minimize all triggers to maximize success. If you don't have the iron-will of DeWayne Johnson, you shouldn't keep foods such as desserts, bread, or other unfriendly snacks.

If you live with others, make sure you talk with and warn them about your new lifestyle changes. If they need to keep some items, find someplace where they can be kept out of sight. This will help everyone who shares your home to understand that you are serious about your new lifestyle. This will lead to a better experience for everyone involved.

Below is a list of foods you need to get rid of and why:

Grains and starches: These foods are very high in carbohydrates. Just a small serving could kick you out of ketosis. You need to eliminate the following:

- Crackers

- Cookies

- Pizza

- Cornstarch

- Beer

- Cornmeal

- Whole Rye

- Brown rice

- Cereals

- Cakes

- Sugar

- Quinoa

- Barley

- Corn

- Wheat

- Pasta

- Rice

Sugary drinks and foods: Sugars have to be avoided at all costs when following the keto diet. Get rid of the following:

- Any product labeled as "low fat"

- Any foods that are processed

- Chocolate

- Sports drinks

- Candy

- Ice cream

- Cakes

- Store-bought smoothies

- Fruit juices

- Maple syrup

- Barley malt syrup

- Dark brown sugar

- Agave nectar

- Molasses

- Sodas

- Light brown sugar

Fruits: Eliminate all fruits that are high in carbs. Dried fruits contain as much sugar as normal fruit but are more concentrated. This makes it easy to eat lots of sugar in a small serving. One cup of raisins has more than 100 grams of carbs, while a cup of grapes only has 15 grams. Get rid of the following:

- Bananas
- Dates
- Grapes
- Mangos
- Apples
- All dried fruits

Legumes and beans: Legumes and beans have moderate amounts of carbs that can damage your keto efforts. Get rid of the following. One cup of beans contains three times the amounts of carbs you should eat in one day. Get rid of the following:

- Edamame
- Navy beans
- Lentils
- Mung beans
- Pinto beans
- Peas
- Black beans
- Kidney beans
- Great northern beans

Processed polyunsaturated oils and fats: Eliminate most seed oil and all oils that say "vegetable." Basically, anything labeled as "partially hydrogenated" or "hydrogenated."

- Vegetable oils
- Margarine

- Cottonseed oil

- Canola oil

- Sunflower oil

- Safflower oil

- Soybean oil

- Hydrogenated oil

Root vegetables: These vegetables contain higher amounts of carbs than other vegetables. Stay away from the following:

- Parsnips

- Sweet potatoes

- Potatoes

Drinks: The worst things to drink when following the keto diet are ones that have hidden sugar or are high in carbs. Here is a list of What You Need to avoid:

- Milkshakes

- Frappuccinos

- Smoothies (unless you make them yourself)

- Sodas

- Sweetened tea

- Vitamin water

- Energy drinks

- Orange juice

- Kombucha tea

- Caffe latte

- Beer

- Soy milk

- Milk

- Vegetable juice

- Coconut water

You might be getting rid of all the unwanted foods in your pantry, but these could feed other people. Please don't just throw these in the trash. Find a homeless shelter or local food pantry to give them to. You will be doing your community a service, plus you have a tax write off.

Go Shopping

Now that you have gotten rid of all the bad foods in your house, it is time to restock your freezer, refrigerator, and pantry with delicious foods that will help you feel great, get healthy and lose weight.

Poultry and meat: You get to eat lots of poultry and meat while following the ketogenic diet. These meats contain no carbs and have vitamin B and essential minerals like potassium, zinc, and selenium. You can eat any of the following meats:

- Deer

- Wild boar

- Bison

- Duck

- Goose

- Lamb

- Chicken

- Turkey

- Bacon

- Sausage

- Ham

- Steak

- Pork

- Beef

Eggs: Eggs are a great option when following a keto diet. They contain less than one gram of carbs and under five grams of protein. Eat them however you like them, such as boiled, scrambled, fried, etc.

Healthy Fats: These are essential for the keto diet and should make up about 75 percent of your total calories. You can use the following fat sources:

- Seeds
- Nuts
- Eggs
- Meat fat
- Fatty fish
- Avocados
- Ghee
- Butter
- Full-fat dairy
- MCT oil
- Extra virgin olive oil
- Olive oil

Seafood and Fish: Fish is a great keto food. They are full of potassium, selenium, vitamin B, and contain almost no carbs. You can get your seafood and fish from the following sources:

- Prawn
- Crayfish
- Scallops
- Lobster
- Crabs
- Mussels

- Oysters

- Shrimp

- Trout

- Mahi-mahi

- Tuna

- Pollock

- Monkfish

- Skate

- Haddock

- Sea bass

- Catfish

- Tilapia

- Cod

- Mackerel

- Anchovies

- Sardines

- Salmon

- Clams

Vegetables: These are the foods you need to eat most while following this diet as long as they are low carb. Vegetables contain fiber, which helps you feel fuller longer. Here is a list of vegetables that you can consume:

- Carrots

- Green beans

- Brussels sprouts

- Peppers

- Kale

- Broccoli

- Cauliflower

- Cabbage

- Zucchini

- Cucumbers

- Eggplant

- Tomatoes

- Olives

- Asparagus

- Avocados

- Lettuce

- Spinach

- Celeriac

- Beets

- Onions

Dairy: You will need to eat these fats in moderation to follow the keto diet successfully. You can get quality fats from high-fat dairy. They also contain minerals, vitamins, and protein. These dairy sources are safe:

- Ricotta cheese

- Plain Greek yogurt

- Swiss cheese

- Cream cheese

- Sour cream

- Cream

- Blue cheese

- Mozzarella cheese

- Gouda cheese

- Cheddar cheese

- Ghee

- Butter

- Paneer

- Feta cheese

- Cottage cheese

Seeds and nuts: These are perfect for the keto diet because they are gut-friendly and dense in nutrients, but these can only be eaten in moderation. Here are some seeds and nut sources:

- Seed milk

- Nut milk

- Sunflower seeds

- Sesame seeds

- Pumpkin seeds

- Hempseeds

- Flaxseeds

- Chia seeds

- Pistachios

- Walnuts

- Pecans

- Macadamia nuts

- Hazelnuts

- Cashews

- Brazil nuts

- Almonds

- Seed oil

- Nut oil

Spices and Seasonings: These are a good way to flavor your meals but you have to be careful as some spices do have some carbs but they shouldn't be a problem if you just learn to eat in moderation. Here is a list of seasonings and spices you can use:

- Oregano

- Thyme

- Rosemary

- Curry

- Nutmeg

- Cloves

- Ginger

- Turmeric

- Cumin

- Cinnamon

- Mustard seeds

- Cayenne pepper

- Chili powder

- Paprika

- Onion powder

- Garlic powder

- Black pepper

- Sea salt

- Cilantro

- Mint

- Basil

- Parsley

Fruits: There are only a few fruits you are allowed to eat while following the keto diet because they are low carb and low in sugar. These have to be eaten in moderation.

- Strawberries

- Blackberries

- Raspberries

- Blueberries

- Lemons

- Limes

The limes and lemons can be used to flavor water or drinks if needed.

Drinks: The following is a list of drinks that are best for you when following a keto diet:

- Tea and Coffee: You can still have your tea and coffee while on the ketogenic diet. Just be sure not to add in any sugar.

- Water: The best thing you can drink for your body is water. Water doesn't have any carbs and replenishes your body of the water it gets rid of. If you want more flavor for your water, try adding in some lemon or drink soda water. If you are going through the keto flu or are having headaches, add some salt to your water.

- Alcohol: You need to be careful when drinking alcohol because some have hidden sugars and carbs. The following alcohols are fine to drink in moderation:

  o Brandy

  o Tequila

  o Vodka

  o Cognac

  o Whiskey

Sweeteners: There are a few low carb natural sugar replacements. You will need to experiment and see what you like the taste of and what your body responds to. When you are having a sugar craving or want to take your coffee to the next level, it is nice to have something on hand to keep your sweet tooth under control and blood sugar stable.

- Stevia

- Erythritol

Getting the Kitchen Ready

Cooking delicious recipes is a great part of the keto diet. It is very easy if you have the correct tools. These tools will help make cooking faster and simpler. Everyone is worth the investment, especially if you cook a lot.

- *Food Scale*

When you are doing your best to reach your macronutrient and caloric goals, a food scale is a necessity. You can to measure any liquid or solid foods and will have the perfect amount each time. If you use it in combination with apps such as MyFitnessPal, you will have the data you need to reach your goals. You can find food scales online for less than $20.

- *Food Processor*

These appliances are crucial for your kitchen arsenal. They are great for processing and blending specific foods together into shakes and sauces. Blenders won't cut it for most foods such as tough veggies like broccoli and cauliflower.

A great blender/processor is the NutriBullet. The containers you use to blend come with drink spouts or lids so you can take them on the go or use them for storage. They are easy to clean and make the entire system very convenient. You can usually find them for around $80 online.

- *Knife Sharpening Stone*

The majority of your time spent in the kitchen is on cutting. You will cut your chopping speed in half if you have a sharp knife. It is also pleasurable to use knives that are sharpened well. Try to sharpen your knives each week to keep them in great shape. Sharpening stones cost less than ten dollars, and you can usually find them online. Most professional chefs will sharpen their knives before each use.

- *Spiralizer*

These fun little gadgets make vegetables into ribbons or noodles in just seconds. They make cooking easier and faster. Noodles have more surface area and only take half the time to cook. This gadget will turn zucchini into zoodles. Add in some marinara or Alfredo sauce, and you will never know that you aren't eating actual pasta. Spiralizers can be found online and in most retail stores. They cost about $30.

- ***Cast Iron Pans***

These beauties have been used for centuries and were some of the first modern cooking utensils. They don't wear out and are healthy to use. They haven't been treated with any chemicals. They retain heat and can go between the stovetop and the oven. They are an easy cleanup. All you need to do is wash them out using a non-scratch sponge and no soap, dry them, and rub them with some oil. This will prevent rust and helps keep them seasoned. Most pans will come pre-seasoned because this method will preserve the coating. They can be found online and in most retail stores. They generally cost between $10 and $80. It all depends on the size and brand. Lodge is still the most popular and continues to be made in the United States.

- ***Electric Hand Mixer***

If you have tried to beat an egg white by hand until they have formed stiff peaks, then you understand how hard this is. Electric hand mixers will save the muscles of your arm, especially if you are mixing heavy ingredients. It can also save you time. You can find good ones online or in retail stores for less than $20.

Meal Prep

Meal prep is the best way to do things if you want to save money, time, and make dieting super easy. Let's learn everything we can about meal prep.

Many people say the hard part of the ketogenic diet is following it. Meal prep can make this a lot easier. Think about a time you might have tried a diet, but you didn't have access to meals. This is why most people turn to fast food places because it is easy and quick. Meal prep turns your refrigerator into a grab-it-and-go dispensary. To simply define meal prep would be the process of planning what you will be eating and how you will make it. The main purpose is saving yourself money and time.

The main part of this is planning and setting aside time to cook. This is a lot easier said than done. Putting forth the effort to plan ahead is going to save energy and time. It will also give you the results that you will be able to feel and see.

More importantly, meal prepping will help you with your dieting goals. It can help you discover the best you by helping you create a constant and healthy routine and stay away from the temptation of eating easy, quick, and unhealthy choices. Having prepped meals in your fridge for easy meals will work wonders for your goals and nutrition. It is hard to be successful when you are dieting as well as trying to maintain a healthy lifestyle since many foods require some sort of prep. We have been hardwired to take the easy route and choose what is convenient and quick.

For some, meal prep might mean chopping veggies beforehand that gets cooked later. It might also mean measuring out ingredients before you start cooking. Most people prepare the meals they will be eating for a whole week in one day and keep them stored in the refrigerator.

Begin Simple

The biggest part of meal prep is making sure it is stress-free and simple. There is no reason that meal prep has to be extravagantly made with complicated ingredients.

Meal Prep Ideas

There are several great ideas when meal prepping. Let's learn about the best ideas out there. You might have to experiment in your kitchen to figure out which way works best for you. This chapter should give you the inspiration you need to create your own meal prep layout.

- *Plan Ahead*

Since you are reading this book, you have likely already decided to try the ketogenic diet. The best way to begin this diet is to start with just a few recipes. You only need enough for one week. Find recipes that you like and make a plan. Create a shopping list and take a trip to the grocery store to get What You Need to make these recipes.

- *Batch Cook*

If you are new to this diet and meal prep, don't let it intimidate you. This way of life is going to save you from stress during the week. Just sit down and plan ahead before you begin cooking. Be patient with yourself when you are trying to multitask in the kitchen. The more you learn to cook many things at one time, the better you will be.

- *Figure Out Your Rhythm*

You might find that you need to sit down with paper and pen and figure out what meals you want to cook. Keep in mind what foods will stay fresher longer along with what foods are on sale at which stores. Put your shopping list in order according to where they are located inside the store. When you have finished your shopping, sit down and figure out how you will attack the prep process. Think about ways to reuse pans or bowls whenever possible. Figure out if you can bake things simultaneously and how you can make the most of your kitchen time. Make sure you have enough time to allow the food to cool before you seal the containers and place them in the fridge.

- *Roast Veggies*

When you need to cook a lot of vegetables, try roasting them all at one time. You could roast a batch of veggies that cook quickly, like mushrooms, cherry tomatoes, and asparagus. You could also make a batch of vegetables that roast slower, like cauliflower, carrots, Brussels sprouts, and broccoli. These can now be stored and used later in the week. This helps reduce time lost and will help you maximize output.

Storage

Here's hoping that meal prep will be a normal routine for your house. For this to happen successfully, you have to choose and invest in the proper storage containers. You need to purchase a few various options like BPA-free plastic, metal, and glass. You can do trial runs to see what works best for you before making a large purchase. Try some and see what you like and what will save you money and time.

Plastic Containers

Quality containers are necessary to keep your food fresh for as long as you can. These are great for meal prep as they are lightweight, freezable, microwavable, and stacks easy. As stated above, be careful with plastics. Make sure they are BPA-free so you won't run the risk of making yourself or your family sick. Plastics aren't biodegradable. This means the earth can't absorb them back into the soil. Plastic can contaminate the soil. Unlike glass, plastics can absorb odors. Whatever you store might taste like what was stored before. Plastic remains cheaper than other storage options, but they don't last as long.

Sectioned Containers: Having these sectioned containers will be a lifesaver. These will give you the space you need to separate each meal item without them being mixed together. You can place the main course in the largest section with the sides in the smaller two. This makes it easy to grab out of the fridge and take with you to work or school to be heated up later.

BPA-free: By now, you have seen or read BPA-free on plastic items, and this is why it is important. BPA are initials for bisphenol-A. This chemical is found in plastics such as consumer goods, food cans, water bottles, and food containers. Researchers say that BPA could seep into beverages and foods from the plastic containers that are made with BPA. Some possible side effects of being exposed to BPA include mental health problems, higher blood pressure, and negative effects on children, infants, and even fetuses.

Stackable: Everybody has a cabinet or drawer full of lids and containers. If you start making meal prep a regular routine, this means you are going to begin accumulating a lot of containers. Having stackable containers will keep your cabinets organized and functional, and this will make your life a lot easier.

Freezer-safe: There will be times when you meal prep and have more food than what you will be able to use in a week. This is why having freezer-safe containers is a necessity. You can also double recipes so you can put them in the freezer to be used later.

Dishwasher-safe: This one should be fairly obvious. Nobody wants to waste time having to hand wash dishes.

Microwave-safe: You are the only person who knows how you like to reheat your meals. Microwaving will be the most convenient. Choosing containers that are microwave-safe is another thing you need to pay attention to.

Glass Containers

Glass containers are great for several reasons. They are environmentally friendly. They are safe to use at various temperatures. This lets you reheat meals in the containers in the oven or microwave. Glass is a bit more expensive than plastic, but you get durability and safety. They also won't keep smells in them after cleaning. Circular, rectangular, or square containers can be found almost anywhere. You need to have a mixture of sizes for more versatility.

Lidded Jars

You need to have a variety of these versatile beauties around. You should try to have several wide-mouth pint and quart jars along with some small four-ounce ones to hold sauces and dressings. They can be used to store healthy salads, snacks, sauces, and soups. Just layer your salad ingredients inside a jar. Don't put the dressing on it, or it will get soggy. This is where those small jars come in handy.

Stainless Steel

These last longer than plastics. Their appearance is nice, and they hold cold and hot temperatures well. They are very durable. They are more expensive, and a drawback is metal can't be used in the microwave.

Skewers

When someone thinks about skewers, they automatically think of kebabs. You can use wooden skewers as a measuring tool for veggies and meats. By doing this, you can cut meat for many skewers and divide them evenly. They can be stored for many days ahead of time. When it is time to cook, just take the meat off the skewers and cook them.

Freeze Smoothies in Muffin Tins

Muffin tins are very useful. To save some time each morning, pour your smoothie into muffin tins. This will save you time and gives you a great smoothie each day. Just take out a few cups, pop them in the blender, and you have a healthy breakfast. Because they are frozen, you don't have to use water or ice.

Keep Records

It is a good idea to keep track of your accomplishments, so you can look back on your achievements. Reaching milestones will give you the encouragement and inspiration to keep pushing forward until you've reached your goals.

Labeling

I used to not worry about labeling my foods as I prepped them until I realized how much I was throwing away. I thought I could remember when everything was bought and would use it before they went bad. Once you begin labeling and prepping meals, you will be more aware of what is in the refrigerator and when you need to use it, and this will, in turn, save you money.

Keep a permanent marker and a roll of freezer tape in the kitchen. Label everything by putting a "best by" date on it, so you know how long every meal is good for.

Thawing

The best way to thaw foods is to put them in the refrigerator. This means you have to think ahead and give yourself time to thaw in the refrigerator before you need it.

Using the cold water method could be quicker than the fridge method, but this requires some attention. The food has to be in a bag that is leak-proof and completely under cold water. The water should be changed every half hour until it is thawed completely.

You should never freeze and thaw fish. It will last for four days in the fridge.

Reheating

Microwaving is the most popular and fastest way to reheat food. I normally try to reheat in one-minute intervals until it is at my desired temperature. Watch the food and stir it after each minute. This makes sure it reaches an even temperature all over.

You could also use your oven or grill to reheat, too. Another option would be using a skillet on the stovetop. You simply empty the meal out into a skillet and stir until it has reached the correct temperature.

When you are reheating leftovers, you need to get them to a temperature of 165.

Storage Tips

When you purchase dairy and meats, always look for products that have a "sell by" date that is the farthest away. It might mean you have to dig to the back, but these foods will stay in storage longer.

Be sure your prepped meals have cooled completely before putting a lid on them and putting them in the freezer or refrigerator. If you put the lid on while it is still hot, it will create steam that will cause the foods to continue to cook. This can cause proteins to become dry and veggies to be overcooked.

Mistakes to Avoid

Now that you understand how to meal prep, let's look at some common mistakes to avoid:

- Don't rush when cooking meals. Thinking about cooking an entire week's meals might seem a bit daunting, but you need to take your time. It is best to prep meals on the weekend or when you have a day off from work.

- Don't leave food on the counter too long, or bacteria might begin forming. Once the food has cooled, you need to keep the food in a lidded container and in the refrigerator to lessen the chances of germs or bacteria setting in.

- Be sure you wash the containers along with their lids after each use. If you don't clean them properly, it could result in bacteria getting into your meals.

- Use fresh ingredients. It is best to prep meals when you get home from the store. If you use vegetables and meats that are old, you might find rotting foods in your refrigerator before you have time to enjoy the meal.

- When you are prepping salad, don't add the salad dressing in. This can cause your vegetables to become soggy. You can add the salad dressing on the bottom and place the protein on top of the dressing. Proteins won't get soggy. You could also put the dressing in a small jar and take it with you.

- Switch up recipes every week or so. This keeps you from getting tired of the same foods. The collection of keto recipes that can be found at the end of this book will make sure you are always excited when it comes time to eat.

- Heat your foods properly. Just be careful not to overheat them as this could cause the food to burn. It can also cause nutrients to become killed off in the reheating process. It could dry out the food where it becomes impossible to eat. If you don't heat it enough, it could leave bacteria in your food that will make you sick.

Meal Prep for Beginners

By now, you understand the basics of a ketogenic diet and meal prepping. As you can see, these two things go hand in hand. These meal prep plans are meant to help make your life easier and lower your stress. This first two-week meal prep plan is perfect for the beginner. It gives you an idea of what your meals should look like and gives you the perfect place to start. It will also slowly introduce you to intermittent fasting.

During the first week, you will have breakfast recipes that you get to enjoy. Then, as you transition into the second week, breakfast recipes will be replaced with keto coffee. Keto coffee doesn't require any prepping, but it only takes a few extra seconds in the morning so it won't ruin your day.

When you start out, the recipes may come off as a bit repetitive, but when you realize how much time you are saving by prepping and not having to constantly figure out your macros, it will be worth it. You will also find shopping lists, which are easy on the wallet. Once you have the big keto staples in your pantry, your shopping trips will cost less. Fats aren't all the same, so you may want to spend a few extra bucks for healthy fats like avocado oil and coconut oil.

The Recipes for WEEK ONE Are:

- Zoodle Chicken Parmesan

- Fajita Salad

- Zucchini Boats

- Breakfast Muffins

The Recipes for WEEK TWO Are:

- Keto Coffee

- Cobb Salad

- Bacon Cheese Burgers

- Chicken Salad Wraps

WEEK ONE Shopping List

Dairy:

- 8-ounce container sour cream
- Cheddar cheese
- Parmesan

Protein:

- 6-ounces cooked ham
- 3 Dozen egg
- 1 pound Italian sausage
- 2-pound flank steak
- 3 bone-in chicken thighs

Produce:

- Tomato
- Broccoli
- Green bell pepper
- Avocado
- 6 zucchinis
- 2 onions
- 3 limes
- 1 head romaine
- Cilantro

Pantry:

- Onion powder

- Garlic powder

- Dijon mustard

- Cooking spray

- Salt

- Red pepper flakes

- 2 cups of pork rings

- Paprika

- Oregano

- 16- ounces Low-carb marinara sauce

- Extra-virgin olive oil

- Cumin

- Coconut oil

- 14.5-ounces chicken broth

- Pepper

Equipment:

- Baking sheet

- Baking dish

- Vegetable spiralizer

- 11 storage containers

- Skillet

- Mixing bowls

- Measuring spoons and cups

- Immersion blender

- Ice tray or silicone molds

- Cutting board
- Knife

Day One:

- Breakfast: Breakfast Muffins
- Lunch: Zoodle Chicken Parmesan
- Dinner: Fajita Salad

Day Two:

- Breakfast: Breakfast Muffins
- Lunch: Fajita Salad
- Dinner: Zucchini Boats

Day Three:

- Breakfast: Breakfast Muffins
- Lunch: Zucchini Boats
- Dinner: Zoodle Chicken Parmesan

Day Four:

- Breakfast: Breakfast Muffins
- Lunch: Fajita Salad
- Dinner: Zucchini Boats

Day Five:

- Breakfast: Breakfast Muffins
- Lunch: Zoodle Chicken Parmesan
- Dinner: Fajita Salad

WEEK ONE Prep

1. Marinate your flank steak.

2. Set your oven to 400.

3. Fix the breakfast muffins and slide them in your oven.

4. Check your breakfast muffins. Once the eggs are completely set, take them out of the oven. Set them aside to cool. Turn the oven to 375.

5. Work through the first four steps of the Zoodle Chicken Parmesan and get your zucchini noodles ready.

6. Work through step five for the Zucchini Boats.

7. In the same skillet you were using for the boats, get the peppers and onions ready for the fajita salad.

8. Check on your chicken, and once it has cooked through, take it out and allow it to cool. Turn the oven to 350 and work through step six of the Zucchini Boats recipe.

9. Once the boats are done, allow them to cool off before placing them in the storage containers.

10. Flip the oven to broiler and follow the second step of Fajita Salad.

11. Finish up the chicken parmesan.

Breakfast Muffins

This recipe makes 5 servings and contains 364 calories; 23 g fat; 30 g protein; 7 g net carbs per serving

What You Need

- Dijon mustard, 1 tsp.
- Diced tomatoes, .5 c
- Shredded cheddar, 1 c
- Cubed ham, 1 c
- Chopped broccoli, 1.5 c
- Garlic powder, .5 tsp.
- Onion powder, .5 tsp.
- Pepper
- Salt
- Eggs, 15
- Cooking spray

What to Do

1. Heat your oven to 400 and grease 15 cups on two muffin tin pans. You can also line them with papers or silicone liners.

2. Mix the garlic powder, onion powder, pepper, salt, and eggs together.

3. Stir in the mustard, tomatoes, cheese, ham, and broccoli.

4. The egg mixture should be evenly poured into the muffin cups.

5. Allow the muffins to bake for 15 minutes. The eggs should be completely set. Allow the muffins to cool off.

6. Place three muffins in five different storage containers.

Fajita Salad

This recipe makes 4 servings and contains 893 calories; 60 g fat; 70 g protein; 11 g net carbs per serving

What You Need

For the Salad:

- Avocado
- Quartered limes, 2
- Shredded cheddar, .5 c
- Sour cream, .5 c
- Chopped romaine, 6 c
- Sliced red and green bell peppers
- Sliced onion
- EVOO, 2 tbsp.

For the Steak:

- Pepper
- Salt
- Chopped cilantro, 1 bunch
- Juice of a lime
- EVOO, .25 c
- Garlic powder, 1 tsp.
- Onion powder, 1 tsp.
- Cumin, 1 tsp.
- Flank steak, 2 lb.

What to Do

For the Steak:

1. Place the flank steak in a bag and add in the pepper, salt, cilantro, lime juice, cumin, onion powder, garlic powder, and oil. Shake everything together and marinate for no more than 24 hours.

2. Once you are ready to cook, flip the broiler on and lay the steak on a baking sheet. Discard the remaining marinade. Bake the steak for three to five minutes on both sides. Allow the steak to rest for at least ten minutes. Thinly slice the steak against the grain.

For the Salad:

1. Heat up a skillet and add in the peppers, onion, and oil. Stir the mixture often, and let it cook for eight to ten minutes, or until the onions turn translucent.

2. In four different storage containers, divide the steak, onions, and peppers. On the other side of the containers, add the cheese, sour cream, lettuce, and lime wedges. Before you serve, top the steak with a quarter of chopped avocado. Mix everything together and squeeze some lime juice over the top.

Zoodle Chicken Parmesan

This recipe makes 3 servings and contains 649 calories; 42 g fat; 45 g protein; 19 g net carbs per serving

What You Need

For Serving:

- Pepper
- Salt
- Low-carb marinara, 1.5 c
- Zucchini noodles, 3 c

For the Zoodles:

- Pepper
- Salt
- Minced garlic, 1 tsp.
- EVOO, 3 tbsp.s
- Zucchini, 4

For the Chicken:

- EVOO, 3 tbsp.
- Garlic powder, 1 tsp.
- Bone-in chicken thighs, 3
- Eggs, 2
- Pepper
- Salt
- Parmesan, .25 c
- Crushed pork rinds, 2 c

What to Do

For the Zoodles:

1. Use a spiralizer to turn the zucchini into noodles.

2. Add the oil to a skillet and cook the garlic for a minute.

3. Add in the zucchini and toss so that it becomes coated in the oil. Allow them to cook for two to five minutes, or until they become tender. Make

sure you don't overcook them because zucchini can quickly become mushy. You want them to have a bit of a crunch.

For the Chicken:

1. Start by placing your oven to 375.

2. Mix the parmesan and pork rinds together in a bowl and add in some pepper and salt. In another dish, beat the eggs.

3. Dry off the chicken and dip each one in the egg wash and then in the pork rind mixture.

4. Use a large pan made of cast iron to warm up the oil and add in the chicken thighs. Cook them for six to seven minutes on each side. Make sure that they cook completely on one side before moving or flipping.

5. Slide the chicken in the oven and let them finish cooking for 25-30 minutes. They should reach 165.

6. In three different containers, add in a cup of zoodles, a half of a cup of marinara, and a chicken thigh.

Zucchini Boats

This recipe makes 3 servings and contains 720 calories; 55 g fat; 44 g protein; 11 g net carbs per serving

What You Need

- Pepper
- Salt
- Parmesan, .75 c
- Chicken broth, 1 c
- Oregano, 2 tsp.
- Minced garlic, 2 tbsp.
- Ground Italian sausage, 1 lb.
- Paprika, 2 tsp.
- Red pepper flakes, 1 tsp.
- Diced onion
- Avocado oil, 1 tbsp.
- Zucchini, 3 – sliced lengthwise

What to Do

1. Heat your oven to 350.

2. Each zucchini half's flesh part should be scooped out using a spoon and then chopped.

3. Add the oil to a skillet and cook the sausage, garlic, and onion until the sausage has brown. This will take about six to eight minutes. Add in the oregano, red pepper flakes, paprika, and zucchini flesh.

4. Add equal portions of the sausage mixture to each of the zucchini shells. Place the zucchini boats in a baking dish and add the broth in the bottom.

5. Top the boats with parmesan and a shake of pepper and salt. Cook boats for 30-35 minutes. The cheese should be bubbly. Place two zucchini boats in each of three different storage containers.

WEEK TWO Shopping List

Dairy:

- 4-ounces blue cheese
- 4-ounces cheddar cheese
- 1-pint heavy cream
- Salted butter

Protein:

- 1 Dozen eggs
- 8-ounces bacon
- 1 ¼ pound skinless and boneless thighs of chicken
- 1 ½ pounds ground beef
- Mayonnaise

Produce:

- Onion
- Parsley
- 2 heads romaine lettuce
- Butter leaf lettuce
- Lemon
- 1 pint grape tomatoes
- Garlic
- 2 cucumbers
- Celery

Pantry:

- Worcestershire sauce

- Salt

- 24-ounces mayonnaise

- Full-fat coconut milk

- Pepper

- Avocado oil

- Apple cider vinegar

Equipment:

- Whisk

- 16 storage containers

- Muffin tin

- Mixing bowl

- Measuring spoons and cups

- Cutting board

- Knife

- 2 baking sheets

Day One:

- Breakfast: Keto Coffee

- Lunch: Bacon Cheese Burger

- Dinner: Cobb Salad

Day Two:

- Breakfast: Keto Coffee

- Lunch: Cobb Salad

* Dinner: Chicken Salad Wraps

Day Three:

* Breakfast: Keto Coffee
* Lunch: Cobb Salad
* Dinner: Chicken Salad Wrap

Day Four:

* Breakfast: Keto Coffee
* Lunch: Chicken Salad Wrap
* Dinner: Bacon Cheese Burger

Day Five:

* Breakfast: Keto Coffee
* Lunch: Bacon Cheese Burger
* Dinner: Cobb Salad

WEEK TWO Prep

1. Start by prepping the Bacon Cheese Burger patties and refrigerate them.

2. Hard-boil the eggs that you need for this week.

3. Place your bacon and chicken thighs on the two baking sheets.

4. Fix your Ranch dressing and place it in the refrigerator.

5. Turn your oven to 375. Slide your bacon and chicken thighs in the oven.

6. Prep the celery, onions, cucumbers, and romaine for the Chicken Salad Wraps and Cobb Salad and place to the side.

7. Check on the things in the oven. Once they are both cooked through, drain the bacon on paper towels and allow the chicken to cool off. The chicken will take longer to cook than the bacon will.

8. Work through the first three steps of the Cobb Salad recipe.

9. Finish out the Bacon Cheese Burger recipe.

10. Pull together the Chicken Salad Wraps.

Ranch Dressing

This recipe makes 1 ½ cups and contains 83 calories; 5 g net carbs per 2 tablespoons; <1 g protein; 7 g fat

What You Need

- Pepper
- Salt
- Mayonnaise, 1 c
- Full-fat coconut milk, .5 c
- Minced garlic, 2 cloves
- Lemon juice, 1 tbsp.
- Apple cider vinegar, 1 tbsp.
- Chopped parsley, 2 tbsp.

What to Do

1. Use a blender to mix all of the ingredients together for one to two minutes, or until it becomes smooth. Taste, and add some pepper and salt if needed.

2. Pour this into a jar and keep it in the refrigerator.

Cobb Salad

This recipe makes 4 servings and contains 545 calories; 38 g fat; 33 g protein; 20 g net carbs per serving.

What You Need

- Ranch dressing, .5 c
- Sliced hard-boil eggs, 4
- Crumbled blue cheese, .5 c
- Chopped cooked bacon, 4 slices
- Chopped onion, .5 c
- Diced cucumbers, 2
- Grape tomatoes, 1 c
- Chopped cooked chicken thighs, 2 c
- Chopped romaine, 2 heads
- Mayonnaise, 1 c

What to Do

1. Place the lettuce evenly in four storage containers.

2. Place the eggs, blue cheese, bacon, onion, cucumbers, tomatoes, and chicken evenly in the four containers on top of the lettuce.

3. Divide the ranch dressing into single-serving containers, two tablespoons per container.

Chicken Salad Wraps

This recipe makes 3 servings and contains 783 calories; 70 g fat; 32 g protein; 2 g net carbs per serving.

What You Need

- Butterhead lettuce, 8 leaves
- Pepper
- Salt
- Mayonnaise, 2 c
- Dijon mustard, 1 tbsp.
- Minced celery, 3 stalks
- Minced onion, 2 tbsp.
- Chopped hard-boil eggs, 6
- Chopped cooked chicken thighs, 1.5 c

What to Do

1. Mix together the mustard, onion, celery, eggs, and chicken. Mix in the mayonnaise. Add in some pepper and salt to your liking.

2. Place the lettuce and egg salad in three storage containers. When you are ready to eat, place the egg salad in the lettuce leaves and wrap up.

Bacon Cheese Burger

This recipe makes 4 servings and contains 772 calories; 6 g net carbs per serving; 61 g protein; 54 g fat.

What You Need

- Grape tomatoes, 1 c
- Chopped avocado
- Chopped romaine lettuce, 1 head
- Pepper
- Salt
- Eggs, 2
- Worcestershire sauce, 1 tbsp.
- Crumbled blue cheese, .5 c
- Crumbled cooked bacon, 4 slices
- Ground beef, 1.5 lbs.

What to Do

1. Mix together the eggs, Worcestershire sauce, blue cheese, bacon, and beef. Add in some pepper and salt. Shape the meat mixture into four patties. Cover them in saran wrap and allow them to refrigerate up to two hours.

2. Heat up your broiler or grill and place the patties on the cooking surface allow them to cook for four to five minutes on both sides. You can cook them to your desired level of doneness. Allow the patties to cool.

3. In four storage containers, add the tomatoes, avocado, and lettuce. Top this with a burger patty.

Keto Coffee

This recipe makes 1 serving and contains 276 calories; 31 g fat; <1 g protein; <1 g net carbs.

What You Need

- Fresh coffee, 8-oz.
- Butter, 1 tbsp.
- Coconut oil, 1 tbsp.
- Heavy cream, 1 tbsp.

What to Do

1. Add all of the ingredients to your blender and mix them together for 30 seconds to a minute. Everything should come together and turn a bit frothy.

Meal Prep for Performance

This next meal prep is designed for the active person. So often, people will use going to the gym as an excuse for eating crap. While it may keep you from gaining weight, and you might drop a few pounds, this isn't the healthiest thing to do. When you are a big gym buff, it can be tough to find time to cook healthy meals. This is where keto meal prep comes in. This meal prep will help you to reduce body fat and maintain all of your lean muscles.

During these two weeks, you will find that the protein intake has been increased, and dairy has been completely eliminated. Dairy will often cause inflammation for people. By reducing or eliminating dairy, you will often see a greater fat reduction. Listen to your body during these two weeks. You may find that your body does better without dairy and higher protein intake. It is also safe to fast while training as long as you make sure you consume some protein close to your workouts.

The Recipes for WEEK ONE:

- Breakfast Pudding

- Spaghetti Squash with Roasted Chicken

- Bratwursts

- Broccoli Stir-Fry

The Recipes for WEEK TWO:

- Keto Coffee

- Salmon and Arugula Salad

- Spaghetti Squash with Bolognese

- Cabbage Stir-Fry

WEEK ONE Shopping List

Protein:

- 4 bone-in chicken thighs
- 1 pound bratwurst sausage
- 1.5 pounds sirloin steak

Produce:

- 4 pound spaghetti squash
- Onion
- Ginger
- 2 crowns broccoli

Pantry:

- Sesame oil
- 16 ounces sauerkraut
- Salt
- Pesto sauce
- Onion powder
- Hemp hearts
- Garlic powder
- Flaxseed
- Shredded coconut
- 5 ounce can full-fat coconut milk
- Coconut aminos
- Cinnamon
- 14.5 ounce chicken broth

- Chia seeds
- Pepper
- Avocado oil
- Sliced almonds
- Vanilla
- Stevia

Equipment:
- Pot
- Mixing bowls
- Measuring spoons and cups
- Cutting board
- Colander
- Knife
- Baking sheet
- Skillet
- 17 storage containers

Day One:
- Breakfast: Breakfast Pudding
- Lunch: Broccoli Stir-Fry
- Dinner: Bratwursts

Day Two:
- Breakfast: Breakfast Pudding
- Lunch: Bratwursts

- Dinner: Spaghetti Squash with Roasted Chicken

Day Three:

- Breakfast: Breakfast Pudding

- Lunch: Spaghetti Squash with Roasted Chicken

- Dinner: Broccoli Stir-Fry

Day Four:

- Breakfast: Breakfast Pudding

- Lunch: Broccoli Stir-Fry

- Dinner: Spaghetti Squash with Roasted Chicken

Day Five:

- Breakfast: Breakfast Pudding

- Lunch: Bratwursts

- Dinner: Broccoli Stir-Fry

WEEK ONE Prep

1. Start to marinate the beef for the <u>Broccoli Stir-Fry</u>.

2. Set your oven to 375 and work through steps two through five for the <u>Spaghetti Squash with Roasted Chicken</u>.

3. As the chicken is cooking, work through the first two steps of <u>Breakfast Pudding</u>.

4. Once your chicken is cooked through, take it out of the oven and let it cool. Turn the heat to 350.

5. After slicing the spaghetti squash in two, the seeds should be removed next. And then, place them on a baking sheet with the cut-side down. Let it bake for 45-50 minutes, or until soft. Once cooked, let it cool and shred the strands out with a fork.

6. Get the <u>Bratwursts</u> ready.

7. Heat up a skillet and boil water in a large pot. Work through the first five steps of Broccoli Stir-Fry.

8. Finish the last steps of Spaghetti Squash with Roasted Chicken.

Breakfast Pudding

This recipe makes 5 servings and contains 397 calories; 5 g net carbs per serving; 7 g protein; 39 g fat

What You Need

- Sliced almonds, .25 c
- Vanilla, 2 tsp.
- Cinnamon
- Salt
- Stevia, 3 tsp.
- Flaxseed, 3 tbsp.
- Shredded coconut, .25 c
- Hemp hearts, .25 c
- Chia seeds, 3 tbsp.
- Unsweetened coconut milk, 2 13.6-ounce cans

What to Do

1. Mix the cinnamon, salt, Stevie, flaxseed, chia seeds, hemp hearts, coconut, and coconut milk together in a pot. Allow this to come to a boil. Next, simmer this over low heat, whisking constantly, until it has thickened. This will take about eight to ten minutes.

2. Remove from the heat. The vanilla should be added next.

3. Divide the pudding between five mason jars and top them with sliced almonds.

Broccoli Stir-Fry

This recipe makes 4 servings and contains 588 calories; 4 g net carbs per serving; 54 g protein; 38 g fat

What You Need

For the Broccoli:

- Pepper
- Sesame oil, .25 c
- Minced garlic, 3 cloves
- Minced ginger, 1 tbsp.
- Coconut aminos, .25 c
- Avocado oil, 2 tbsp.
- Trimmed and separated broccoli, 2 crowns
- Salt, 1 tsp.

For the Marinade:

- Sliced sirloin steak, 1.5 lb.
- Pepper
- Salt
- Sesame oil, 2 tbsp.
- Garlic powder, 1 tsp.
- Onion powder, 1 tsp.
- Avocado oil, .25 c
- Coconut aminos, 6 tbsp.

What to Do

In a mixing container, combine together all the ingredients for the marinade. Add in the steak and toss. Make sure that the steak is completely coated. Allow the steak to marinate for at least 30 minutes.

For the Broccoli:

1. Fill up a pot halfway with water and add in a teaspoon of salt. Let this come to a boil.

2. Place the broccoli in the water and blanch for one to three minutes. Pour into a colander to drain. Rinse the broccoli with cold water so that it doesn't continue to cook. Place to the side.

3. Add the ginger, garlic, and avocado oil to a large skillet and let them all cook for 30 seconds.

4. Mix in the beef. Discard the marinade. Cook the beef, stirring constantly, for two to three minutes. Mix in the sesame oil, coconut aminos, and broccoli. Add in some pepper and salt. Continue to cook this mixture until the beef has reached your desired doneness.

5. Split this mixture between four storage containers.

Bratwursts

This recipe makes 4 servings and contains 525 calories; 42 g fat; 24 g protein; 8 g net carbs per serving

What You Need

- Pepper
- Salt
- Garlic powder, 1 tsp.
- Chicken broth, 1.5 c
- Sauerkraut, 16-ounces – drained
- Bratwurst, 1 lb.
- Sliced onion
- Avocado oil, 2 tbsp.

What to Do

1. Add the oil, bratwurst, and onion to a cast iron skillet. Allow this to cook for six to eight minutes, or until they get some color.

2. Mix in the pepper, salt, garlic powder, broth, and sauerkraut. Let this mixture simmer for 30-40 minutes. The sausages should be cooked all the way through.

3. In four containers, add a cup of sauerkraut and one bratwurst.

Spaghetti Squash with Roasted Chicken

This recipe makes 4 servings and contains 361 calories; 6 g net carbs per serving; 18 g protein; 30 g fat

What You Need

- Pesto, .25 c
- Cooked spaghetti squash
- Pepper
- Salt
- EVOO, .25 c
- Garlic powder, 1 tsp.
- Onion powder, 1 tsp.
- Bone-in chicken, 4 3-ounce thighs

What to Do

1. Set your oven to 375.

2. Dry off the chicken thighs and lay them in a shallow dish.

3. Add in the onion powder, garlic powder, and oil, along with some pepper and salt. Mix everything and make sure that the chicken is coated.

4. On a baking sheet, lay the chicken out.

5. Bake the chicken for about thirty to forty minutes. Cook the chicken thoroughly until it reaches 165 degrees.

6. Toss the pesto and the cooked spaghetti squash together. Season it with some pepper and salt. Make sure that the squash is completely coated.

7. Place the noodles evenly in four containers and top each one with a thigh. Let everything cool off before you place on the lids.

WEEK TWO Shopping List

Protein:

- 3 4-ounce salmon fillets
- 2 ½ pounds ground beef

Produce:

- 4 pound spaghetti squash
- 4 scallions
- Onion
- Lemon
- Garlic
- Celery
- Head of cabbage
- Green bell pepper
- 8 ounces of arugula

Pantry:

- 14.5-ounce can diced tomatoes; low-sugar
- 6-ounce can tomato paste
- Salt
- Oregano
- Garlic salt
- Garlic powder
- Extra-virgin olive oil
- Coconut oil
- Coconut aminos
- Pepper
- Apple cider vinegar

Equipment:

- 11 storage containers
- Skillet
- Measuring cups and spoons
- Cutting board
- Knife
- Baking sheet baking dish

Day One:

- Breakfast: Keto Coffee or Fasting
- Lunch: Cabbage Stir-Fry
- Dinner: Salmon and Arugula Salad

Day Two:

- Breakfast: Keto Coffee of Fasting
- Lunch: Spaghetti Squash with Bolognese
- Dinner: Cabbage Stir-Fry

Day Three:

- Breakfast: Keto Coffee or Fasting
- Lunch: Salmon and Arugula Salad
- Dinner: Spaghetti Squash with Bolognese

Day Four:

- Breakfast: Keto Coffee or Fasting
- Lunch: Cabbage Stir-Fry
- Dinner: Salmon and Arugula Salad

Day Five:

- Breakfast: Keto Coffee of Fasting

- Lunch: Spaghetti Squash with Bolognese

- Dinner: Cabbage Stir-Fry

WEEK TWO Prep

1. Get the vegetables ready for the Spaghetti Squash with Bolognese and Cabbage Stir-Fry.

2. Set your oven to 450 and work through the first three steps of the Salmon and Arugula Salad.

3. Once the salmon is cooked through, take it out of the oven and lower the oven down to 350. Finish putting together the salmon salad.

4. Slice the spaghetti squash lengthwise and clean out the seeds. In a casserole dish, the squash should be laid with its cut-side down and pour water about a quarter inch. Allow the squash to cook for 45-50 minutes. Take the squash out of the oven and allow it to cool. With a fork, scrape out the strands from the squash.

5. Work through the first four steps of the Spaghetti Squash with Bolognese recipes.

6. Heat up your skillet and work through the first four steps of the Cabbage Stir-Fry recipe.

Cabbage Stir-Fry

This recipe makes 4 servings and contains 550 calories; 33 g fat; 49 g protein; 8 g net carbs per serving

What You Need

- Chopped scallions, 4
- Coconut aminos, 2 tbsp.
- Apple cider vinegar, 2 tbsp.
- Salt
- Pepper
- Chopped cabbage, 1 head
- Minced garlic, 2 cloves
- Ground beef, 1.5 lb.
- Coconut oil, 1 tbsp.

What to Do

1. In a skillet, the oil should be heated up before adding the garlic and beef. Brown the beef.

2. Add in the cabbage and let the mixture cook for eight to ten minutes more. The cabbage should wilt slightly.

3. Mix in the vinegar and coconut aminos. Season with a little bit of pepper and salt.

4. Divide the stir-fry between four storage containers. Serve the stir-fry with some scallions. You can also top it with some toasted sesame oil, sriracha, and sesame seeds if you want.

Spaghetti Squash with Bolognese

This recipe makes 4 servings and contains 415 calories; 24 g fat; 33 g protein; 18 g net carbs per serving

What You Need

- Cooked spaghetti squash
- Pepper
- Diced tomatoes, 14.5-ounce can – drained
- Erythritol, 1 tbsp.
- Oregano, 1 tbsp.
- Garlic powder, 1 tsp.
- Salt
- Tomato paste, 2 tbsp.
- Ground beef, 1 lb.
- Chopped bell pepper
- Chopped celery, 2 stalks
- Chopped onion
- EVOO, 1 tbsp.

What to Do

1. Add the oil to a skillet. Mix in the bell pepper, celery, and onion. Cook them, stirring often, for six to eight minutes. Once the vegetables have cooked, mix in the ground beef. Cook until the meat is thoroughly cooked.

2. Add in the pepper, salt, garlic powder, oregano, erythritol, tomatoes, and tomato paste. Boil the mixture before simmering it for 20-30 minutes. Stir the mixture occasionally.

3. Allow the sauce to cool.

4. Place the cooked spaghetti squash in equal amounts in four containers and top each of them with the Bolognese.

Salmon and Arugula Salad

This recipe makes 3 servings and contains 393 calories; 4 g net carbs per serving; 26 g protein; 31 g fat

What You Need

- Arugula, 4.5 c
- Juice of a lemon
- Garlic salt, 1 tsp.
- EVOO, 5 tbsp. – divided
- Salmon, 3 4-ounce fillets

What to Do

1. Set your oven to four hundred and fifty degrees. On a baking sheet, place the foil.

2. Rub the salmon fillets with two tablespoons of oil and season with the garlic salt. Lay the salmon on the baking sheet and drizzle the lemon juice over top of them.

3. Bake the salmon for 8-12 minutes, or until it flakes easily. Allow the salmon to rest for ten minutes.

4. In three containers, add 1.5 cups of arugula and season with some pepper and salt. Top with the salmon. When you are ready to eat, drizzle with a tablespoon of oil and toss everything together.

Meal Prep for Maintenance

After you have achieved your weight loss goals, keeping that weight off tends to be the hardest part. Your protein and calories will be upped with this meal prep, but your carbohydrate intake will remain low. When you hit the maintenance period, keeping your carbs low is still the most important thing. Calories and protein intake don't have to be stressed over as much.

Your body now runs on fat, so you can play around and see how your body works in ketosis. If you do want to try out some more carbs, pick sources that are unprocessed. Carbs are best consumed right after you have exerted a lot of energy. Stay far away from processed or refined carbs, though. Make sure you listen to what your body has to say. Give your body the carbs that it wants.

Recipes for WEEK ONE:

- Frittata

- Chili

- Salmon Salad

- Meatloaf with Green beans

Recipes for WEEK TWO:

- Keto Coffee

- Chicken Legs with Rice

- Taco Salad

- Caesar Salad

WEEK ONE Shopping List

Dairy:

- Parmesan
- 1 pint heavy cream
- Crumbled feta cheese
- Shredded cheddar

Protein:

- 1 pound sausage
- 4 6-ounce salmon fillets
- 8 ounces ground pork
- Dozen eggs
- 1 pound ground beef
- 8 ounces bacon

Produce:

- Spinach
- Scallions
- 1 pint raspberries
- Mixed greens
- 1 pound green beans
- Celery
- 6 ounces broccoli florets
- Red bell pepper

Pantry:

- Worcestershire sauce

- Walnuts

- 16 ounce can tomato paste

- 15-ounce can diced tomatoes

- Salt

- Pork rinds

- Pecans

- Ketchup

- 4-ounce can diced green chiles

- Garlic salt

- EVOO

- Erythritol

- Cumin

- Chili powder

- Coconut oil

- Pepper

- 14.5 ounce can beef broth

- Apple cider vinegar

- Mustard

Equipment:

- 18 storage containers

- Slow cooker

- Skillet

- Mixing bowls

- Measuring spoons and cups

- Cutting board
- Knife
- Baking sheet

Day One:

- Breakfast: Breakfast Frittata
- Lunch: Salmon Salad
- Dinner: Meatloaf with Green Beans

Day Two:

- Breakfast: Breakfast Frittata
- Lunch: Chili
- Dinner: Meatloaf with Green Beans

Day Three:

- Breakfast: Breakfast Frittata
- Lunch: Chili
- Dinner: Salmon Salad

Day Four:

- Breakfast: Breakfast Frittata
- Lunch: Salmon Salad
- Dinner: Chili

Day Five:

- Breakfast: Breakfast Frittata
- Lunch: Salmon Salad

- Dinner: Meatloaf with Green Beans

WEEK ONE Prep

1. Set your oven to 400 and work through steps one through five for the Meatloaf with Green Beans. Clean out the bowl and reuse it for the Frittata.

2. Using a cast iron skillet, cook the meats for the chili. First, brown the ground beef, and then set to the side. Next, cook the bacon, and set to the side. Finally, brown up the sausage for the frittata and the chili.

3. Prep all of the fresh produce for the Frittata and the celery for the chili. Place to the side.

4. Check the meatloaf, and once it is cooked through, take out of the oven and let it cool. Lower the heat of the oven to 375.

5. Work through the first two steps for the Chili.

6. In the skillet you used for the meats, work through steps three through six for the Frittata.

7. Boil water and a dash of salt to a large pot. Add in the green beans and cook them for three to four minutes. Drain off the beans and place them in ice water to stop the cooking. Drain and follow the sixth step of the Meatloaf recipe. Place a square of butter on top of the beans in their containers.

Frittata

This recipe makes 5 servings and contains 392 calories; 31 g fat; 23 g protein; 5 g net carbs per serving

What You Need

- Thinly sliced scallions, 3
- Shredded cheddar, .5 c – divided
- Pepper
- Salt
- Heavy cream, 2 tbsp.
- Beaten eggs, 8
- Spinach, 2 c
- Chopped red bell pepper
- Chopped broccoli florets, 1 c
- Ground sausage, 8 oz.

What to Do

1. Set your oven to 375.

2. Add the sausage to a cast iron skillet and brown for four to five minutes. Take the sausage out of the skillet and drain off all but a tablespoon of fat.

3. Put the bell pepper, spinach, and broccoli in the skillet and cook until the spinach wilts. This will take about two to three minutes. Mix the sausage back in.

4. Whisk the cream and eggs together with some pepper and salt. Pour the eggs over the sausage mixture. Stir in a quarter cup of cheddar cheese until everything is combined.

5. Slide this into the oven. Bake for about half an hour. The tops should be browned. Take the frittata out of the oven and top with the rest of the cheese. Put this under the broiler until the cheese has melted and crisped up.

6. Allow the frittata to cool and then slice it into five equal wedges. Place each wedge into five storage containers. Sprinkle on the scallions.

Meatloaf with Green Beans

This recipe makes 4 servings and contains 481 calories; 27 g fat; 49 g protein; 10 g net carbs per serving

What You Need

- Blanched green beans, 3 c
- Erythritol, 1 tbsp.
- Apple cider vinegar, 1 tbsp.
- Ketchup, .25 c
- Pepper
- Salt
- Mustard, 1 tsp.
- Heavy cream, .25 c
- Parmesan, .25 c
- Crushed pork rinds, .5 c
- Egg
- Ground pork, 8 oz.
- Ground beef, 8 oz.

What to Do

1. 400 degrees should be your oven's temperature. On a baking sheet, place a foil.

2. Mix together the mustard, cream, parmesan, pork rinds, egg, pork, and beef. Add in some pepper and salt.

3. Form the meat into a loaf shape and place it on the baking sheet.

4. Mix together the erythritol, vinegar, and ketchup. Brush this over the meatloaf.

5. Slide this into the oven. Bake for thirty-five to forty minutes. Ensure it has a temperature of 160 degrees.

6. Allow the meatloaf to cool before slicing it into four equal pieces.

7. Place ¾ of a cup of green beans and a slice of meatloaf into four storage containers.

Salmon Salad

This recipe makes 4 servings and contains 456 calories; 34 g fat; 36 g protein; 7 g net carbs per serving

What You Need

- Crumbled feta, .25 c
- Fresh berries, .25 c
- Salad greens, 4 c
- Erythritol, 1 tbsp.
- Coconut oil, 1 tbsp.
- Whole pecans, .5 c
- Pepper
- Salt
- EVOO, 2 tbsp.
- Salmon fillets, 4 6-oz. fillets

What to Do

1. Preheat your broiler and line a cooking sheet with foil.

2. Use olive oil to rub the salmon. Drizzle with some pepper and salt. Lay them on the cooking sheet and allow them to broil for 8-12 minutes. The salmon should easily flake with a fork.

3. Take the salmon out and set to the side.

4. Meanwhile, add the erythritol, coconut oil, and pecans to a skillet. Stir until the erythritol has dissolved and the pecans have become fragrant. This will take three to five minutes. Take the pecans out of the skillet and set them to the side.

5. Toss together the feta, berries, and greens in a large bowl.

6. Using four storage containers, add a heaping cup of salad mix in each and top with a salmon fillet and two tablespoons of pecans.

Chili

This recipe makes 5 servings and contains 629 calories; 37 g fat; 46 g protein; 20 g net carbs per serving

What You Need

- Worcestershire sauce, 1 tbsp.
- Chili powder, 1 tbsp.
- Cumin, 1 tbsp.
- Garlic salt, 1 tsp.
- Pepper, 1 tsp.
- Shredded cheese
- Sour cream
- Diced green chiles, 4 oz.
- Tomato paste, 6 oz.
- Diced tomatoes with juices, 15 oz.
- Chopped celery, 1 c
- Beef broth, 1 c
- Cooked ground sausage, 8 oz.
- Diced cooked bacon, 8 oz.
- Cooked ground beef, 8 oz.

What to Do

1. Add everything except for the sour cream and shredded cheese to a crockpot. Mix everything together. Set the cooker to high for four to six hours, or you can set it to low for eight to ten hours.

2. Allow the chili to cool off, and then divide evenly into five containers. Serve with some sour cream and cheese.

WEEK TWO Shopping List

Dairy:

- 8 ounce sour cream
- Salted butter
- Parmesan
- Heavy cream
- Cheddar cheese

Protein:

- Dozen eggs
- 12 ounces boneless skinless chicken thighs
- 6 chicken legs
- Pound ground beef

Produce:

- 2 limes
- Head romaine
- Lemon
- 1 pint grape tomatoes
- Garlic
- Head cauliflower
- Head cabbage
- 2 onions

Pantry:

- Mustard

- Worcestershire sauce

- Taco seasoning

- Low-carb salsa

- Onion powder

- Garlic salt

- EVOO

- 16 ounce can black olives

- 14.5 ounce can beef broth

- Anchovy paste

Equipment:

- 3 storage containers

- Skillet

- Mixing bowl

- Measuring spoons and cups

- 7 16-ounce mason jars

- Cutting board

- Knife

Day One:

- Breakfast: Keto Coffee or Fasting

- Lunch: Taco Salad

- Dinner: Chicken Legs with Rice

Day Two:

- Breakfast: Keto Coffee of Fasting

- Lunch: Caesar Salad

- Dinner: Taco Salad

Day Three:

- Breakfast: Keto Coffee or Fasting

- Lunch: Chicken Legs with Rice

- Dinner: Caesar Salad

Day Four:

- Breakfast: Keto Coffee or Fasting

- Lunch: Caesar Salad

- Dinner: Taco Salad

Day Five:

- Breakfast: Keto Coffee of Fasting

- Lunch: Caesar Salad

- Dinner: Chicken Legs with Rice

WEEK TWO Prep

1. Set your oven to 375. Rub the chicken thighs with onion and garlic powder, pepper, and salt. Bake the chicken for twenty to thirty minutes.

2. Boil a pot of water and cook the eggs.

3. Work through the first step of Taco Salad.

4. As the chicken and beef are cooking, prep your cauliflower rice.

5. Once the chicken thighs are cooked through, remove and allow to cool. Once the ground beef is browned, allow it to cool as well.

6. Get the ingredients for the Taco Salad and Caesar Salad prepared.

7. Work through steps four through seven for the Chicken Legs.

8. As the chicken is cooking, put together the salads. Work through the first two steps for the Caesar Salad and the second step for the Taco Salad.

9. Once the chicken legs are cooked through, place them on a plate and allow to cool. Follow steps one through three of Chicken Legs with Rice to prepare the rice.

10. Once everything has cooled, divide the rice and chicken legs between four containers.

Caesar Salad

This recipe makes 4 servings and contains 586 calories; 6 g net carbs per serving; 33 g protein; 50 g fat

What You Need

- Chopped romaine, 1 head
- Chopped cooked chicken thighs, 2 c
- Parmesan, .5 c
- Sliced hard-boil eggs, 4
- Thinly sliced onion, .5 c
- Grape tomatoes, 1 c
- Low-carb Caesar dressing, .75 c

What to Do

1. Add three tablespoons of dressing to the bottom of four mason jars.

2. Next, add in the tomatoes, onion, eggs, cheese, and chicken. Top with the lettuce. When you are ready to eat, shake everything together and enjoy.

Taco Salad

This recipe makes 3 servings and contains 931 calories; 65 g fat; 57 g protein; 22 g net carbs per serving

What You Need

- Lime wedges, 2 limes
- Shredded cabbage, 1 head
- Shredded cheddar, .75 c
- Sliced black olives, 16 ounces
- Grape tomatoes, 1 c
- Low-carb salsa, .75 c
- Beef broth, .5 c
- Taco seasoning, .25 c
- Ground beef, 1 lb.

What to Do

1. Add the ground beef to a skillet and cook until browned through. This will take about seven to ten minutes. After adding the taco seasoning and the broth, simmer it until it has thickened, about three to five minutes. Make sure that beef has cooled completely before making the salad.

2. Using three mason jars, divide out the salsa, sour cream, tomatoes, olives, cheese, beef, cabbage, and a lime wedge. It needs to be layered in that order. When you are ready to eat, squeeze in the lime juice and shake the salad together.

Chicken Legs with Rice

This recipe makes 3 servings and contains 502 calories; 35 g fat; 34 g protein; 10 g net carbs per serving

What You Need

- Pepper
- Chicken legs, 6
- Onion powder, 1 tbsp.
- Garlic salt, 1 tbsp.
- Salt
- Shredded cheddar, .5 c
- Heavy cream, .5 c
- Uncooked cauliflower rice, 3 c
- Salted butter, 4 tbsp. – divided
- Chopped onion

What to Do

1. Cook the onion in two tablespoons of butter in a large skillet. The onions should become translucent. This will take about five minutes.

2. Mix in the cauliflower, and let it cook for five minutes.

3. Stir in the cream cheese along with some pepper and salt. Mix until the cheese has melted. This will take about two to three minutes. Pour this into another dish and allow it to cool off.

4. Using the same skillet, add in the reaming butter.

5. Rub the chicken with pepper, garlic salt, and onion powder.

6. For fifteen minutes, cook the chicken in a pan. Turn the meat frequently. The skin should be golden and has reached 165.

7. Using three storage containers, add in a cup of rice and two chicken legs.

Breakfast

Breakfast Casserole

This recipe makes 12 servings and contains 285 calories; 23 g fat; 17 g protein; 2 g net carbs per serving

What You Need

- Shredded Swiss cheese, 1 c
- Pepper
- Salt, .5 tsp.
- Heavy cream, 1 c
- Beaten eggs, 9
- Chopped onion
- Bulk breakfast sausage, 1 lb.

What to Do

1. Set your oven to 350 and grease a 9" x 13" casserole dish.

2. Add the sausage to a skillet and cook. Crumble up the sausage as it cooks. Allow it to brown up. This will take about five minutes.

3. Mix in the onions. Cook for two to three more minutes, or until the onions soften. Set this off of the heat.

4. As the sausage cools off, beat together the pepper, salt, cream, and eggs.

5. Fold the cheese and sausage into the eggs.

6. Spread the mixture into your greased casserole dish.

7. Slide this into the oven and allow it to back for an hour.

8. Cool the casserole slightly before you slice it into 12 pieces.

9. If meal prepping, place a square of the casserole into 12 storage containers.

10. These will keep for five days in the refrigerator or for six months in the freezer. To reheat, place them in the oven at 350 for 20 minutes. You can also thaw in the fridge and microwave for a couple of minutes.

Breakfast Pizza

This recipe makes 4 servings and contains 644 calories; 47 g fat; 43 g protein; 10 g net carbs per serving

What You Need

- Halved cherry tomatoes, 8
- Shredded mozzarella, .5 c
- Red pepper flakes
- Oregano, 1 tsp.
- Heavy cream, .25 c
- Beaten eggs, 8
- Sliced mushrooms, 1 c
- Chopped onion, .5
- Cubed pancetta, 8 oz.
- Unsalted butter, 2 tbsp.

What to Do

1. Heat up your broiler and move the rack to the highest position.

2. Using an ovenproof pan, add the butter and cook until it starts to bubble. Add in the pancetta, stirring occasionally, until it turns brown. This will take about three to five minutes.

3. Mix in the mushrooms and onion. Stir often. Cook for three mins or until the vegetables become soft. Spread this across the bottom of the pan.

4. Whisk the red pepper flakes, oregano, cream, and eggs together. Pour the mixture into the hot pan. Cook the eggs, without stirring them, so that they set around the edges. To pull back the eggs' edges, use a spatula. Tilt the eggs and let the uncooked eggs to run into the empty spot. Cook until the edges have set up again.

5. Sprinkle the eggs with the cheese and then top with the tomatoes. Slide the frittata in the oven under the broiler and cook until the cheese has melted and browned. This will take about three to five minutes.

6. Allow the frittata to cool and then slice it into four wedges.

7. For meal prepping, place a wedge of the frittata into four storage containers.

8. These will keep for five days in the fridge or six months in the freezer. Allow them to rest in the fridge overnight to thaw and then microwave for

a couple of minutes. You can also heat them in the oven at 375 for five to ten minutes.

Baked Eggs in Avocado

This recipe makes 6 servings and contains 613 calories; 6.07 g net carbs per serving; 21 g protein; 56 g fat

What You Need

- Pepper
- Salt
- Shredded cheddar, 6 tbsp.
- Eggs, 6
- Lime juice, 4 tbsp.
- Avocados, 3

What to Do

1. Start by placing your oven to 450.

2. Carefully slice open each avocado, remove the pit and some of the flesh.

3. Put the avocados onto a baking sheet. Brush each half with lime juice.

4. Crack one egg into each avocado half.

5. Season with pepper and salt.

6. Put into the oven and bake for ten minutes.

7. Carefully remove from oven and sprinkle with cheese. Bake for another two to three minutes to melt the cheese.

8. Using six storage containers, add one avocado. Cool completely before placing into the refrigerator.

9. This will keep for three days in the refrigerator. This won't freeze well because of the avocado.

Ham and Cheese Waffles

This recipe makes 6 servings and contains 538 calories; 1.33 g net carbs per serving; 46 g protein; 39 g fat

What You Need

- Basil, .5 tsp.
- Chopped ham, .25 c
- Baking powder, 1 tsp.
- Pepper, .25 tsp.
- Salt, .5 tsp.
- Paprika, .5 tsp.
- Shredded cheddar, .25 c
- Melted butter, .75 c
- Eggs, 8

What to Do

1. Using two bowls, separate the whites and yolks of four eggs. Keep the other four eggs to the side.

2. Into the bowl holding the egg yolks, add in the baking powder, butter, and salt. Whisk until thoroughly combined.

3. Fold in the cheese and ham gently.

4. Into the bowl holding the egg whites, whisk these until stiff peaks form.

5. Place half the whites into the yolk mixture, fold gently, and let sit for a few minutes.

6. After adding in the remaining egg whites, fold to incorporate.

7. Add some batter to a greased waffle maker. Cook for four minutes.

8. Continue with the rest of the batter until all is used up.

9. Using six storage containers, add a waffle into each. Cool completely before closing.

10. These can be frozen for up to six months or kept in the refrigerator for five days.

Bacon, Egg, and Cheese Casserole

This recipe makes 8 servings and contains 307 calories; 37.8 g fat; 25.5 g protein; 4.1 g net carbs per serving

What You Need

- Pepper
- Salt
- Chopped green onions, 3
- Minced garlic, 2 cloves
- Chopped onion, 1
- Heavy whipping cream, .5 c
- Sour cream, .75 c
- Shredded cheddar, 1.5 cups
- Eggs, 12
- Sliced bacon, 12

What to Do

1. Start by placing your oven at 350.

2. Put the bacon into a skillet and cook until crispy. When cooked, put onto paper towels to drain. Once drained and cooled a bit, crumble into bits.

3. Add the pepper, salt, whipping cream, sour cream, and eggs into a bowl. Whisk until thoroughly incorporated.

4. Grease a 9" x 13" casserole dish with olive oil. Add the shredded cheese onto the bottom and spread until even.

5. Pour the egg mixture on top and then top with the bacon bits.

6. Wrap the top with aluminum foil.

7. Put into the oven and bake for 35 minutes until the edges are browned and the middle is set.

8. Take out of the oven. Garnish with green onions.

9. Cut into eight equal pieces.

10. Using eight storage containers, add in one portion per container.

11. This will keep for five days in the refrigerator. You can also freeze it up to six months. To reheat, allow it thaw in the fridge and microwave for a few minutes.

Blackberry Egg Bake

This recipe makes 4 servings and contains 163 calories; 1 g net carbs per serving; 9.83 g protein; 12 g fat

What You Need

- Salt
- Zest of one orange
- Coconut or almond flour, 4 tbsp.
- Vanilla, .25 tsp.
- Melted butter, 1 tbsp.
- Chopped rosemary, 1 tsp.
- Grated ginger, 1 tsp.
- Blackberries, .5 c
- Eggs, 6

What to Do

1. Start by placing your oven at 350.

2. Take four ramekins and grease them with olive oil.

3. Add salt, orange zest, coconut flour, ginger, butter, vanilla, and eggs into a bowl. Stir until combined. The batter should be smooth.

4. Add in rosemary and stir to combine.

5. Evenly divide the batter into the four ramekins.

6. Put the ramekins onto a baking sheet and divide the blackberries evenly among the ramekins.

7. Place the baking sheet into the oven and bake for 20 minutes until eggs are done.

8. Carefully remove from oven and let cool slightly before serving.

9. Let the ramekins cool completely. Gently remove from ramekins and place into four storage containers.

10. These can be frozen for six months or refrigerated for five days.

Mushroom and Sausage Frittata

This recipe makes 6 servings and contains 388 calories; 3.47 g net carbs per serving; 29 g protein; 16 g fat

What You Need

- Butter, 1 tbsp.
- Salt, .5 tsp.
- Pepper, .5 tsp.
- Paprika, .25 tsp.
- Basil, .5 tsp.
- Greek yogurt, .5 c
- Chopped onion, 1 medium
- Sliced mushrooms, 1 c
- Shredded cheddar, 1 c
- Chopped kale, 6 oz.
- Eggs, 12
- Breakfast sausage, 1 lb.

What You Need

1. Start by placing your oven to 350.

2. Place a large ovenproof skillet onto your stove and warm on medium heat.

3. Put the sausage into the skillet and cook until done or no longer pink. Spoon it out onto paper towels and let drain. Set to the side.

4. Add butter into the same skillet and melt. When melted, add the mushrooms and onions into the skillet. Sauté until the onions are translucent. Stir frequently. Remove and set to the side.

5. Put the basil, paprika, pepper, salt, yogurt, and eggs into a large bowl. Whisk until completely combined.

6. Add in the onion, mushrooms, half of the cheese, kale, and sausage. Stir again to combine everything.

7. Add more butter and pour this mixture into the same skillet. Cook on medium heat. Cook for four minutes. Do not stir.

8. Take off from the heat and sprinkle on the rest of the cheese.

9. Bake in the oven until the center is done or for about thirty minutes. Take out of the oven and let it cool for a few minutes before slicing.

10. Slice into six equal triangles and place into six storage containers.

11. This can be refrigerated for five days or frozen for six months.

Spinach and Leek Eggs

This recipe makes 6 servings and contains 238 calories; 5.7 g net carbs per serving; 13 g protein; 18 g fat

What You Need

- Shredded cheddar, 1.5 c
- Eggs, 6
- Minced garlic, 2 cloves
- Chopped leeks, 2
- Spinach, 1 c
- Pepper, .25 tsp.
- Salt, .25 tsp.
- Chili powder, 1 tsp.
- Coconut oil, 2 tbsp.

What to Do

1. Start by placing your oven to 425.

2. Place a skillet on medium heat onto the stove and warm. Melt the coconut oil.

3. Put in the spinach, garlic, and leeks. Sauté for eight minutes until soft.

4. The eggs should be cracked in a bowl. Add in the chili powder, pepper, salt, and cheese. Stir to combine.

5. Pour into skillet and scramble the eggs until the desired doneness.

6. Using six storage containers, divide evenly and allow to cool completely before placing into the refrigerator for five days or freeze for six months.

Chorizo Bake

This recipe makes 4 serving, and contains 432 calories; 37 g fat; 26 g protein; 5.07 g net carbs per serving

What You Need

- Pepper
- Salt
- Chopped bell pepper, 1
- Chopped onion, 1 small
- Sliced bacon, 2
- Chopped chorizo sausage, 6 oz.
- Sour cream, 2 tbsp.
- Almond milk, 2 tbsp.
- Eggs, 4
- Coconut oil, 1 tbsp.

What to Do

1. You need to warm your oven to 350.

2. Over medium heat, warm a large skillet on the stove. Cook the bacon. Make sure it is crispy. Drain the bacon onto paper towels after removing it from the skillet.

3. Add coconut oil to the skillet and let it melt. Add in bell pepper and onion. Cook for six minutes until slightly browned.

4. Add in the chorizo and continue to cook.

5. Place the sour cream, almond milk, and eggs into a large bowl and whisk until combined. Season with pepper and salt.

6. Pour into skillet and lower heat. Sprinkle with bacon and let it cook until the center is set.

7. Cut into four servings.

8. Using four storage containers, add one section into each container. Refrigerate for five days or freeze for six months.

Mushroom and Spinach Muffins

This recipe makes 12 servings and contains 173 calories; 13 g fat; 4.2 g protein; .8 g net carbs per serving

What You Need

- Italian seasoning, .5 tsp.
- Garlic powder, 1 tsp.
- Pepper
- Salt
- Chopped spinach, 2 c
- Chopped mushrooms, 1 c
- Coconut milk, .5 c
- Shredded cheese, 1 c
- Eggs, 8

What to Do

1. You need to warm your oven to 350.

2. Grease a muffin tin with olive oil.

3. Into a bowl, add garlic powder, Italian seasoning, pepper, salt, coconut milk, cheddar cheese, and eggs. Whisk to combine.

4. Add in the spinach and mushrooms.

5. Divide this mixture out into the muffin tin.

6. For twenty minutes, bake in the preheated oven until thoroughly cooked.

7. Take out of the oven and let cool.

8. For food prep, allow it to cool completely and place into individual storage containers for five days or freeze for six months.

Lemon Poppy Pancakes

This recipe makes 4 servings and contains 378 calories; 5 g net carbs per serving; 31.3 g protein; 27.1 g fat

What You Need

- Erythritol, .25 c
- Liquid stevia, 10 drops
- Salt, .25 tsp.
- Coconut flour, .5 c
- Protein powder, 1 scoop
- Poppy seeds, 2 tbsp.
- Baking powder, 1 tsp.
- Heavy cream, 1 tbsp.
- Ricotta, 6 oz.
- Eggs, 6
- Zest and juice of 2 lemons

What to Do

1. In a food processor or blender, put the juice and zest of one lemon, stevia, eggs, and ricotta. Process until smooth.

2. Pour into a large bowl. Add in the protein powder, flour, poppy seeds, salt, and baking powder. Stir to combine.

3. Put a large nonstick skillet onto the stove and warm on medium heat.

4. Place about one-fourth cup of the batter into the skillet.

5. Cook until bubble form on top and sides are set. Gently turn over and cook on the other side until browned.

6. Place onto plates and continue with batter until all is gone.

7. In another bowl, put the zest and juice of the other lemon, erythritol, and heavy cream. Whisk until combined.

8. Drizzle this lemon glaze over pancakes and enjoy.

9. Place any uneaten pancakes into a storage container and place into the freezer for up to six months or in the fridge for three days.

Coconut Blueberry Porridge

This recipe makes 4 servings and contains 392 calories; 11.53 g net carbs per serving; 11 g protein; 21 g fat

What You Need

- Ground flaxseed, .5 c
- Blueberries, 1 c
- Ground cinnamon, 1 tsp.
- Ground nutmeg, .5 tsp.
- Vanilla, 1 tsp.
- Salt
- Coconut flour, .5 c
- Grated coconut, .5 c
- Coconut milk, 2 c

What to Do

1. Place a saucepan on the stove on low heat. Pour in the coconut milk.

2. Whisk in the salt, nutmeg, cinnamon, flaxseed, and flour. Increase the heat and cook until it is just bubbling.

3. Add in the vanilla and continue to cook until as thick as you want it.

4. Spoon into bowls and top with blueberries.

5. Divide into four storage containers. Once completely cooled, place into refrigerator for five days.

Egg Cups with Hollandaise

This recipe makes 6 servings and contains 428 calories; 42 g fat; 9 g protein; 2 g net carbs per serving

What You Need

- EVOO, .25 c
- Cayenne
- Salt, .5 tsp.
- Zest and juice of a lemon
- Hot water, .5 c
- Halved avocado
- Pepper
- Eggs, 6
- Bacon, 6 slices

What to Do

1. Set your oven to 400.

2. Place the bacon in the bottom of six cups of a cupcake tin. Sprinkle in some pepper.

3. Let the bacon bake for ten minutes.

4. Take the bacon out of the oven and then carefully crack an egg into each c.

5. Place this back in the oven and let it cook for ten more minutes, or until the eggs are cooked to your desired doneness.

6. Meanwhile, add the cayenne, salt, lemon zest and juice, hot water, and avocado to a blender. Blend the mixture until it forms a smooth consistency. You may want to pause and scrape down the sides a time or two.

7. As the blender is running, drizzle in the oil until it is completely incorporated. Evenly divide the sauce between six storage containers.

8. Once the eggs have finished cooking, carefully take them out of the muffin tin.

9. Place an egg into six storage containers. When you are ready to serve, drizzle with the hollandaise sauce.

10. The hollandaise and egg cups need to be stored in separate containers in the fridge. The hollandaise will last a couple of days, so it is best to make it on demand. The egg cups will last in the fridge for four days.

Asparagus Breakfast Muffins

This recipe makes 6 servings and contains 411 calories; 31 g fat; 27 g protein; 7 g net carbs per serving

What You Need

- Pepper
- Salt, .5 tsp.
- Rosemary, 1 tsp.
- Dijon, 1 tsp.
- Heavy cream, .25 c
- Beaten eggs, 10
- Shredded Swiss cheese, 1 c
- Trimmed asparagus cut into bite-sized chunks, 1 lb.
- Chopped onion, .5
- Chopped bacon, 8 oz.
- Unsalted butter, 4 tbsp.
- EVOO or coconut oil – for greasing

What to Do

1. Prepare a 12-c muffin tin and then grease them. Set to 375 degrees the temperature of your oven.

2. Add the butter to a large skillet and cook until it starts to bubble. Put in the bacon and cook until it has browned. This will take about five minutes.

3. Mix in the asparagus and onion. Stir occasionally. Cook until they become tender or for approximately five minutes

4. Spoon this into the muffin cups.

5. Sprinkle with cheese.

6. Mix together the pepper, salt, rosemary, mustard, cream, and eggs.

7. In the muffin cups, pour in the egg mixture.

8. Cook this in the oven for 12-15 minutes, or until the eggs are completely cooked through. Take these out and carefully take the muffins out of the tin. Using six storage containers, add two muffins. Allow them to cool completely before covering the containers.

9. This will keep in the fridge for three days or will freeze for up to six months. Place them in the fridge overnight to thaw and then microwave

for a couple of minutes. You can also slide them in the oven at 375 for ten minutes.

Tex-Mex Scramble

This recipe makes 4 servings and contains 508 calories; 40 g fat; 32 g protein; 5 g net carbs per serving

What You Need

- Shredded cheddar, .5 c
- Beaten eggs, 8
- Minced garlic, 2 cloves
- Minced jalapeno
- Chopped scallions, 6
- Bulk chorizo, 8 oz.

What to Do

1. Add the chorizo to a large skillet and cook until it has browned up. Make sure that you break the chorizo up as you go. This will take about five minutes.

2. Add in the jalapeno and scallions. Stir the mixture occasionally, until softened. This will take about an extra three minutes.

3. Mix in the garlic.

4. Add in the eggs.

5. Cook the mixture, scrambling the eggs as they cook through.

6. Sprinkle in the cheese. Stir everything together.

7. For meal prepping, divide the eggs between four containers.

8. This will keep in the refrigerator for three days, or you can freeze them up for six months. To thaw them out, let them rest in the fridge overnight and then microwave for a couple of minutes.

Egg Stuffed Peppers

This recipe makes 4 servings and contains 459 calories; 6 g net carbs per serving; 33 g protein; 34 g fat

What You Need

- Parmesan, .5 c
- Red pepper flakes
- Pepper
- Salt, .5 tsp.
- Italian seasoning, 1 tsp.
- Heavy cream, .25 c
- Beaten eggs, 8
- Sliced mushrooms, 4 oz.
- Bulk Italian sausage, .5 lb.

What to Do

1. Start by heating your oven to 400.

2. On a baking sheet, place the peppers with the cut-side up. Bake them for five minutes, or until they have softened up.

3. Meanwhile, add the sausage to a large skillet and cook until browned, breaking the meat up as it cooks. This will take about five minutes.

4. Mix in the mushrooms. Stir occasionally until the mushrooms become soft. This will take another five minutes. Let this cool slightly.

5. Beat the red pepper flakes, pepper, salt, Italian seasoning, cream, and eggs together.

6. Fold the cooled mushrooms and sausage into the egg mixture.

7. Divide this mixture between the pepper halves and top them with the cheese.

8. Place this back in the oven. Allow the peppers to cook until the eggs have set and the cheese on top has browned. This will take about 40 minutes. Allow the peppers to cool off before storing.

9. Place one stuffed pepper half in four containers.

10. These will keep for five days in the fridge or six months in the freezer. Thaw them in the refrigerator overnight and then microwave them for a

couple of minutes. You can also heat them in the oven at 400 for 30 minutes.

Pancakes

This recipe makes 6 servings and contains 518 calories; 40 g fat; 13 g protein; 15 g net carbs per serving

What You Need

- Salt
- Baking soda, 2 tsp.
- Erythritol, 1 tbsp.
- Coconut flour, 1 c
- Vanilla, 1 tsp.
- Beaten eggs, 8
- Heavy cream, 1 c
- Melted butter, 1 c

What to Do

1. Whisk the vanilla, eggs, cream, and butter together.

2. Whisk the salt, baking soda, erythritol, and coconut flour together in a separate bowl.

3. In the coconut flour mixture, pour the egg mixture and stir together until it just comes together.

4. Brush some of the melted butter onto a heated skillet.

5. Cook a quarter of a cup of the batter onto the pan until bubbles start to form on the top. This will take about two minutes.

6. Flip the pancake, and cook for a couple of minutes more.

7. Continue this process until you use up all of the pancake batter. It should make 18 pancakes.

8. Using six storage containers, place three pancakes into each.

9. These will keep for five days in the refrigerator and will keep in the freezer for six months. Let them thaw overnight in the refrigerator and heat in the microwave for a minute. You can also bake them at 350 for five to ten minutes.

Main Dishes

Keto Lasagna

This recipe makes 12 servings and contains 554 calories; 43 g fat; 29 g protein; 9 g net carbs per serving

What You Need

- Shredded mozzarella, 3 c – divided
- Sliced salami, 16 oz.
- Whole-milk ricotta, 16 oz.
- Pesto, 7 oz.
- Bulk Italian sausage, 1 lb.
- Italian seasoning, 1 tsp.
- Crushed tomatoes, 2 14-oz. cans – drain the juices off of one can
- Minced garlic, 6 cloves
- Minced shallot
- Avocado oil, .25 c

What to Do

1. Start by placing your oven to 350.

2. In a large skillet, heat the oil until it simmers.

3. Add in the shallow and let it cook for two minutes. Make sure you stir often. Cook in the garlic, stirring constantly, and until it smells delicious.

4. Mix in the tomatoes, as well as the juices of one can, and the Italian seasoning. Let this come up to a simmer. Let this cook, stirring occasionally, for five minutes.

5. Meanwhile, place the sausage in a large skillet and cook until browned. Make sure you break the sausage up as it cooks. This will take about five minutes. Take this off the heat and set to the side.

6. Mix together the ricotta and pesto.

7. Prepare a casserole dish with a 9"x13" size. In its bottom, pour in the sauce about one-half c.

8. Place a layer of salami over the sauce and then smooth over a layer of the ricotta mixture. Pour a dash of 1 c mozzarella on top. Add a quarter to a half of a cup of the meat mixture over the top. Place on another layer of salami and another layer of ricotta, and top with a cup of mozzarella.

9. Place one last layer of salami over the top and cover with the rest of the sauce. Top with the rest of the mozzarella.

10. Place this on a rimmed baking sheet in case the lasagna boils over. Place this in the oven and let it bake for an hour. Let the lasagna cool slightly, and then slice it into 12 pieces.

11. Place a square of lasagna into 12 storage containers.

12. The lasagna will keep refrigerated for five days or frozen for six months. Reheat the lasagna at 350 for 45 minutes.

Cabbage and Pork Stir-Fry

This recipe makes 6 servings and contains 698 calories; 4 g net carbs per serving; 54 g protein; 50 g fat

What You Need

- Chili oil, .5 tsp.
- Sesame oil, .5 tsp.
- Soy sauce, 1 tbsp.
- Juice of 2 limes
- Minced garlic, 3 cloves
- Freshly grated ginger, 1 tbsp.
- Shredded cabbage, 2 c
- Sliced scallions, 6
- Ground pork, 1 lb.
- Coconut oil, 3 tbsp.

What to Do

1. Pour the coconut oil into a large frying pan and let it heat up until it starts to shimmer.

2. Add in the pork and cook until it browns up. Break it apart as it cooks. This will take about five minutes.

3. Place the ginger, cabbage, and scallions. Stir constantly and cook until the vegetables have softened up. This will take about three minutes.

4. Cook the garlic next until they all smell delicious.

5. Mix in the chili oil, sesame oil, soy sauce, and lime juices. Cook the mixture for one to two minutes, or until everything is heated.

6. Divide the mixture between six containers.

7. This will keep in the refrigerator for three days or will last for six months in the freezer. Thaw them in the fridge overnight and microwave a couple of minutes to heat through.

Glazed Meatloaf

This recipe makes 6 servings and contains 265 calories; 15 g fat; 24 g protein; 2 g net carbs per serving

What You Need

- Pepper
- Salt
- Balsamic vinegar, 1 tbsp.
- Eggs, 2
- Parmesan cheese, .33 c
- Almond flour, .5 c
- Chopped mushrooms, 1 c
- Chopped parsley, 2 tbsp.
- Minced garlic, 4 cloves
- Chopped onion, 1
- Chopped bell pepper, 1
- Ground beef, 3 lbs.
- Glaze Ingredients:
- Stevia, 1 tbsp.
- Balsamic vinegar, 2 c
- Zero-sugar ketchup, .25 c

What to Do

1. You need to warm your oven to 375.

2. Place all the ingredients for the meatloaf into a large bowl. Hand-mix all of the ingredients so that they are combined thoroughly.

3. Place the mixture into a 13" x 9" casserole dish and shape into an oval loaf.

4. Put into the oven and bake for 30 minutes.

5. To make the glaze, put the stevia, balsamic vinegar, and ketchup into a small saucepan on medium heat. Stir until combined. Make sure it doesn't boil.

6. Carefully take out of the oven and spread the glaze on top.

7. Bake in the oven again for another twenty mins.

8. Carefully remove and let cool for a few minutes.

9. Slice any unused portion and place into storage containers. Place into the freezer for six months or in the fridge for five days.

Thai Beef

This recipe makes 6 servings and contains 226 calories; 19 g fat; 19 g protein; 2 g net carbs per serving

What You Need

- Pepper
- Salt
- Chopped green onion, 3
- Chopped bell pepper, 1
- Lemon pepper, 1.5 tsp.
- Beef broth, 1 c
- Peanut butter, 4 tbsp.
- Beefsteak, 1 pound
- Olive oil, 2 tbsp.
- Coconut aminos, 1 tbsp.
- Onion powder, .25 tsp.
- Garlic powder, .25 tsp.

What to Do

1. Into a bowl, add the lemon pepper, coconut aminos, beef broth, and peanut butter. Mix well to combine.

2. Slice up the steak into strips.

3. Put a large skillet onto the stove on medium and warm up two tablespoons of olive oil.

4. When heated, add in the steak, garlic powder, onion powder, pepper, and salt. Sauté for seven minutes.

5. Add in the bell pepper and cook for an additional three minutes.

6. Pour in the peanut butter mixture and onions. Cook for an additional two minutes, stirring frequently.

7. Using six storage containers, evenly divide. Store in the refrigerator for five days or freeze for six months.

Meatballs and Mushroom Sauce

This recipe makes 6 servings and contains 436 calories; 26 g fat; 32 g protein; 2 g net carbs per serving

What You Need

- Meatball Ingredients:
- Chopped parsley, 1 tbsp.
- Coconut flour, .75 c
- Beef broth, .25 c
- Coconut aminos, 1 tbsp.
- Garlic powder, 1 tsp.
- Pepper
- Salt
- Chopped jalapeno, 1
- Chopped onion, 1
- Ground beef, 2 lbs.
- Mushroom Sauce Ingredients:
- Pepper
- Salt
- Beef broth, .5 c
- Sour cream, .25 c
- Coconut aminos, 1 tsp.
- Chopped onions, 1 c
- Sliced mushrooms, 2 c
- Olive oil, 2 tbsp.
- Butter, 2 tbsp.

What to Do

1. You need to warm your oven to 375.

2. Take a baking sheet and line it with parchment paper.

3. In a large dish, place the entire meatball ingredients. Using your hands, mix until all ingredients are combined well.

4. Form into meatballs and place onto prepared baking sheet.

5. Put into the oven and bake for 20 minutes.

6. Place a saucepan on medium heat and warm the olive oil.

7. When heated, add mushrooms and cook for four minutes, stirring frequently.

8. Add onions and cook for an additional four minutes.

9. Add in the beef stock, sour cream, and coconut aminos. Stir well to combine. Cook until everything is warmed through.

10. Take off heat and season with pepper and salt.

11. Take the meatballs out of the oven and drizzle mushroom sauce over the meatballs.

12. Divide evenly into storage containers and either place into the refrigerator for five days or freeze for six months.

Roasted Pork Belly

This recipe makes 6 servings and contains 367 calories; 2 g net carbs per serving; 31 g protein; 38 g fat

What You Need

- Cored and wedged apples, 3
- Pepper
- Salt
- Chopped parsley, 2 tbsp.
- Garlic, 4 cloves
- Chopped onion, 1
- Scored pork belly, 2 lbs.
- Stevia, 2 tbsp.
- Lemon juice, 1 tbsp.
- Olive oil, 3 tbsp.

What to Do

1. Put the apples, pepper, salt, parsley, garlic, onion, one cup of water, lemon juice, and stevia into a blender. Process until almost smooth.

2. Place the pork belly into a steamer tray and steam for one hour. Take out of the steamer and set to the side.

3. You need to warm your oven to 425.

4. Take three tablespoons of olive oil and rub over pork. The apple mixture should be poured on top of the pork.

5. Put into a preheated oven for 30 minutes or until cooked through.

6. Allow to cool.

7. Slice the pork and divide into six containers, place into the refrigerator for five days or freeze for six months.

Lamb Meatballs

This recipe makes 4 servings and contains 286 calories; 2 g net carbs per serving; 21 g protein; 24 g fat

What You Need

- Pepper
- Salt
- Paprika, .5 tsp.
- Shredded cheddar, .25 c
- Egg, 1
- Garlic powder, .5 tsp.
- Onion powder, .5 tsp.
- Coconut flour, .5 c
- Ground lamb, 1.5 lb.

What to Do

1. You need to warm your oven to 400.

2. Take a baking sheet and line it with parchment paper.

3. Place the pepper, salt, paprika, onion powder, garlic powder, egg, cheese, coconut flour, and lamb into a large bowl. Using your hands, mix until thoroughly combined.

4. Shape into meatballs and put onto the prepared baking sheet.

5. Put into the oven and bake for 15 minutes.

6. Divide evenly into storage containers and place into the refrigerator for five days or in the freezer for up to six months.

Mushroom Pork Chops

This recipe makes 4 servings and contains 599 calories; 4 g net carbs per serving; 30 g protein; 13 g fat

What You Need

- Pepper
- Salt
- Mayonnaise, 1 c
- Chopped onion, 1
- Minced garlic, 2 cloves
- Sliced mushrooms, 1.5 c
- Coconut oil, 4 tbsp.
- Balsamic vinegar, 1 tbsp.
- Pork chops, 4

What to Do

1. You need to warm your oven to 350.

2. Place a large skillet onto the stove on medium heat and melt two tablespoons coconut oil. Add in the onion, mushrooms, and garlic. Sauté for four minutes. Take off heat and set to the side.

3. Sprinkle the pork chops with pepper and salt.

4. Add the rest of the coconut oil to the skillet. When heated, add the pork chops and brown on each side.

5. Place into a baking dish and put into the oven. Bake for 30 minutes.

6. When done, remove the pork chops carefully and set them to the side.

7. Place a saucepan on medium heat. Add in the mushroom mixture, mayonnaise, and balsamic vinegar. Stir until everything is combined. Take off heat.

8. Drizzle the sauce over pork.

9. Using four storage containers, add one pork chop to each. Store in the refrigerator for five days or freezer for six months.

Zesty Halibut

This recipe makes 4 servings and contains 581 calories; 4 g net carbs per serving; 38 g protein; 46 g fat

What You Need

- Pepper, .25
- Salt, .25
- Olive oil, 2 tbsp.
- Chopped onions, .25 c
- Lime juice, 2 tbsp.
- Avocados, 2
- Chopped cauliflower, 1 head
- Boneless halibut, 4 6-oz. fillets

What to Do

1. Pulse the cauliflower in a food processor until it resembles rice.

2. Add a tablespoon of oil to a skillet. Cook the rice until it has become tender or for about eight minutes. Take the rice out and set it to the side.

3. In a clean food processor, mix the onion, lime juice, and avocado until smooth.

4. Add the rest of the oil to the skillet.

5. Rub the fish with pepper and salt. You can also add on any other spices that you would like.

6. Place the fish in the skillet, working in batches if you need to, and cook four to five minutes on each side.

7. Once the fish is cooked through, place a fillet in four storage containers and divide the cauliflower rice between the four bowls. Divide the avocado sauce between four single-serving dressing cups. When ready to enjoy, drizzle the sauce over everything and serve.

8. This cannot be frozen. It will last five days in the refrigerator.

Bok Choy Stir-Fry

This recipe makes 4 servings and contains 68 calories; 1 g net carbs per serving; 3 g protein; 6 g fat

What You Need

- White pepper, .5 tsp.
- Fish sauce, 1 tsp.
- Sliced red bell pepper
- Sliced leeks, 2
- Minced garlic, 4 cloves
- Coconut oil, 2 tbsp.
- Coconut aminos, 2 tbsp.
- Sliced shitake mushrooms, 1 c
- Chopped bok choy, 4 c

What to Do

1. Add the coconut oil to a skillet and once heated, add in the mushrooms, bell pepper, garlic, and leeks. Cook the vegetables until they have softened up. Stir occasionally.

2. Add in the bok choy and cook for another four minutes. Stir occasionally.

3. Mix in the pepper, fish sauce, and coconut aminos. Let this cook for another minute.

4. Divide the stir-fry between four storage containers.

5. You can keep it for five days in the refrigerator. You can also freeze it up to six months. To reheat, let it thaw overnight and then add it to a skillet to heat through.

Chicken Quesadilla

This recipe makes 4 servings and contains 599 calories; 41 g fat; 53 g protein; 8 g net carbs per serving

What You Need

- Pepper, .25 tsp.
- Salt, .5 tsp.
- Sliced avocados, 1
- Low-carb wraps, 4
- Grilled chicken breasts, 4
- Favorite shredded cheese, 1 c
- Minced jalapeno, 4 tsp.

What to Do

1. Place one of the low-carb wraps on the frying pan. Cook the wrap for two minutes on each side and then sprinkle a quarter cup of the cheese over the wrap. Place a shredded chicken breast, a teaspoon of jalapeno, and some avocado slice to one have of the wrap.

2. Carefully fold the wrap over the chicken and flatten it out.

3. Take the wrap out and continue with the other three wraps.

4. Place one wrap in a storage container.

5. This will keep for five days in the fridge and up to six months in the freezer. To reheat, let it thaw overnight in the refrigerator and then warm in the oven for ten minutes at 350.

Spinach and Artichoke Chicken

This recipe makes 4 servings and contains 450 calories; 2 g net carbs per serving; 39 g protein; 24 g fat

What You Need

- Pepper, .5 tsp.
- Chopped onion, .5
- Minced garlic, 2 cloves
- Salt, 1 tsp.
- Parmesan, .5 c
- Spinach, 2.5 c
- Chopped artichoke hearts, 2.5 c
- Cream cheese, 4 oz.
- Shredded mozzarella, .5 c
- Boneless skinless chicken breasts,

What You Need

1. Start by placing your oven to 400.

2. Grease a casserole dish and rub the chicken pepper and salt.

3. After placing the chicken in the casserole dish, bake for thirty minutes.

4. As the chicken is cooking, mix together the garlic, cream cheese, parmesan, spinach, onions, and artichokes. Make sure the mixture is well combined.

5. When the 30 minutes are up, carefully take the casserole dish out of the oven. Slice a pocket in the middle of each of the chicken breasts.

6. Divide the artichoke mixture between the four chicken breasts, stuffing it inside of the pocket.

7. The shredded mozzarella should then be sprinkled over the chicken.

8. Bake it again in the oven for an additional fifteen minutes.

9. Check to make sure the chicken reached 165.

10. Once done, allow it to cool off before placing a chicken breast in a storage container.

11. This will keep in the refrigerator for five days. You can also freeze it for up to six months. To reheat, let it thaw in the refrigerator and then microwave it for a couple of minutes.

Chicken Soup

This recipe makes 4 servings and contains 381 calories; 3 g net carbs per serving; 31 g protein; 23 g fat

What You Need

- Chopped celery, .5 c
- Sour cream, .5 c
- Pepper, 1 tsp.
- Shredded chicken, 2 c
- Cream cheese, 4 oz.
- Butter, 3 tbsp.
- Salt, 1 tsp.
- Chicken stock, 4 c

What to Do

1. Add the sour cream, pepper, salt, butter, cream cheese, and chicken stock to a blender and mix until everything is well combined.

2. Pour this into a large pot. Add in the chicken, carrots, and celery.

3. Once the mixture boils, simmer it on low heat. Let it cook for a few minutes until everything has heated through.

4. Divide the soup between four bowls.

5. This will keep for five days in the refrigerator, or you can freeze it for up to six months. When you want to reheat it, let the soup thaw in the refrigerator overnight and then add to a pot to heat it through.

Lamb Goulash

This recipe makes 6 servings and contains 287 calories; 3 g net carbs per serving; 11 g protein; 12 g fat

What You Need

- Ground lamb, 1.5 lbs.
- Cauliflower florets, 2 c
- Chicken broth, 1.5 cups
- Diced tomatoes, 1 14.5 oz. can
- Tomato paste, 1 tbsp.
- Chopped onion, 1
- Chopped red bell pepper, 1
- Chopped bell pepper, 1
- Water, 1.5 c
- Salt
- Pepper

What to Do

1. On medium heat, place a large pan. The ground lamb should be added next. Cook until no longer pink.

2. Add in the bell peppers and onion. Continue to cook for another four minutes, stirring frequently.

3. Add in the water, diced tomatoes, and cauliflower. Give everything a good stir and allow it to simmer.

4. Place a lid on the skillet and cook for five minutes.

5. Add in seasonings and tomato paste and stir well to combine.

6. Take off heat and allow to cool. Cool completely and transfer to storage containers. Store in the refrigerator for five days or in the freezer for six months.

Mediterranean Pork

This recipe makes 4 servings and contains 241 calories; 1 g net carbs per serving; 28 g protein; 19 g fat

What You Need

- Pepper, 1 tsp.
- Salt, 1 tsp.
- Minced garlic, 4 cloves
- Greens of choice, 4 c
- Chopped zucchini
- Halved cherry tomatoes, 1 c
- Rosemary, 4 tsp.
- Olive oil, 4 tbsp.
- Bone-in pork chops, 4

What to Do

1. Start by placing your oven at 425.

2. Rub the pork chops with the oil, pepper, garlic, salt, and rosemary.

3. Place them on a baking sheet and slide into the oven. Let the pork chops bake for ten minutes.

4. Turn the heat down to 350 and let them continue to cook for 25 minutes. Remove the chops and let them cool off before storing.

5. Meanwhile, toss together the greens, zucchini, and tomatoes.

6. In four storage containers, divide out the salad mixture and add in one pork chop.

7. This will keep for five days in the refrigerator.

Slow Cooker Chili

This recipe makes 8 servings and contains 466 calories; 36 g fat; 31 g protein; 4 g net carbs per serving

What You Need

- Sour cream, 1 c
- Shredded cheddar, 1 c
- Salt, 1 tsp.
- Cumin, 1 tsp.
- Garlic powder, 1 tsp.
- Ground coriander, 1 tsp.
- Chili powder, 3 tbsp.
- Chopped onion
- Boneless pork shoulder cut into cubes, 2 lbs.

What You Need

1. Place everything except for the sour cream and cheese in your slow cooker and stir everything together.

2. Place the lid on the cooker and set it to low for eight hours or on high for four hours.

3. Once the chili is done, allow it to cool and add 1 ½ cups of chili into eight storage containers. When you are ready to serve, top with some sour cream and cheese.

4. This will keep for five days in the refrigerator or six months in the freezer. Allow the chili to thaw overnight in the fridge and then microwave for a couple of minutes. You can also reheat on the stovetop, stirring occasionally, until it has heated through. You can add in a little broth if the chili is too thick.

Slow Cooke Stew

This recipe makes 8 servings and contains 933 calories; 66 g fat; 69 g protein; 6 g net carbs per serving

What You Need

- Pepper, .25 tsp.
- Salt, 1 tsp.
- Rosemary, 1 tsp.
- Thyme, 1 tsp.
- Dijon, 1 tbsp.
- Garlic powder, 2 tsp.
- Dry red wine, 1 c
- Chopped celery, 4 stalks
- Bag frozen pearl onion, 8 oz.
- Halved or quartered button mushrooms, 1 lb.
- Chopped onions, 2
- Stew meat cut into cubes, 1 ½ lb.

What to Do

1. Add all of the ingredients to your slow cooker and stir everything together.

2. Place on the lid and set your cooker to low for eight hours or on high for four hours. Allow the stew to cool off.

3. Add 1 ½ cups of stew to eight storage containers.

4. The stew will last for five days in the refrigerator or for six months in the freezer. Allow this to thaw overnight in the refrigerator and then microwave for a couple of minutes. You can also heat it through on the stovetop. You can add in some broth if it is too thick.

Burrito Bowls

This recipe makes 4 servings and contains 528 calories; 35 g fat; 41 g protein; 12 g net carbs per serving

What You Need

- Chopped avocado
- Sour cream, .5 c
- Shredded cheddar, 1 c
- Cooked cauliflower rice, 2 c
- Sliced bell pepper
- Slice onion
- Pork belly, 1 lb.
- Minced scallions, 6
- Minced garlic, 6 cloves
- Salt, .5 tsp.
- Minced jalapeno
- Juice of 3 limes
- Chopped cilantro, 1 bunch
- Avocado oil, .5 c – divided

What You Need

1. Mix together the scallions, garlic, salt, jalapeno, lime juice, cilantro, and a quarter cup of oil. Reserve two tablespoons of the mixture.

2. Add the rest of the mixture to a baggie and add in the pork belly. Shake it around so that the pork gets coated. Seal up the bag and allow it to be refrigerated for four to eight hours.

3. Heat up the remaining oil in a large skillet until it starts to shimmer.

4. Take the meat out of the marinade and wipe away the excess. Place the meat in the oil, cooking until it reaches 145. This will take about five minutes on each side. Place this on a plate and tent it with foil.

5. Using the same skillet, add in the bell pepper and onion. Occasionally stir the veggies. Cook for about five minutes, or until they become soft.

6. Thinly slice the meat against the grain and add it back into the pan. Mix in the reserved marinade. Cook the meat mixture for two more minutes, or until everything is coated with the marinade.

7. Divide the meat and veggies between four storage containers. In four other containers, add ½ cup of the cauliflower rice. When you are ready to eat, mix the rice and meat mixture and top with the avocado, sour cream, and cheese.

8. These will keep for five days in the refrigerator. Reheat them for a couple of minutes in the microwave.

Chicken Casserole

This recipe makes 8 servings and contains 609 calories; 56 g fat; 25 g protein; 9 g net carbs per serving

What You Need

- Shredded cheddar, 1 c
- Cream of mushroom soup, 10.5 oz. can
- Bag frozen pearl onions, 8 oz.
- Halved button mushrooms, 1 lb.
- Bone-in chicken thighs, 8

What to Do

1. Start by setting your oven to 350.

2. Place the chicken thighs into the bottom of a 9" x 13" casserole dish. Add in the onions and mushrooms. Make sure that they are mixed up but scattered across the pan.

3. Mix the cheese and soup together and pour the mixture over the chicken.

4. Cover the dish with aluminum foil and bake it for an hour and 15 minutes, or until the chicken has reached 165 and the juices run clear. Allow this to cool.

5. In eight storage containers, place a chicken thigh along with some of the vegetables and sauce.

6. This will keep for six months in the freezer and three days in the refrigerator. Allow it to thaw overnight in the fridge and then reheat it for a couple of minutes in the microwave. You can also bake it for 20-30 minutes at 375.

Tuna Casserole

This recipe makes 9 servings and contains 761 calories; 59 g fat; 53 g protein; 9 g net carbs per serving

What You Need

- Shredded cheddar, 1 c
- Oil-packed tuna, 1 lb. – drained
- Dijon, 1 tbsp.
- Dried dill, 1 tsp.
- Zest of a lemon
- Cream of mushroom soup, 10.5 oz. can
- Minced garlic, 3 cloves
- Sliced zucchini, 2
- Chopped onion
- Avocado oil, .25 c

What to Do

1. Start by placing your oven to 350.

2. Add the oil to a large skillet and heat it until it shimmers. Add in the zucchini and onion, stirring occasionally, and cook until they start to soften up. This will take about five minutes.

3. Mix in the garlic and cook for about 30 seconds, or until it becomes fragrant. Take this off of the heat and let it cool.

4. Mix together the mustard, dill, lemon zest, and mushroom soup. Whisk it until smooth. Stir in the cooled veggies, cheese, and tuna. Stir well.

5. Spread this into a 9" x 13" casserole dish. Bake the casserole until it is bubbly, around an hour. Allow the casserole to cool.

6. Divide the casserole between nine storage containers.

7. This will keep for three days in the refrigerator and six months in the freezer. Let it thaw in the refrigerator overnight and microwave for a couple of minutes. You can also bake it for 15-20 minutes at 375.

Fettuccine Alfredo

This recipe makes 6 servings and contains 691 calories; 62 g fat; 29 g protein; 8 g net carbs per serving

What You Need

- Pepper
- Parmesan, 1 c
- Heavy cream, .5 c
- Butter, 8 tbsp.
- Cream cheese, 8 oz.
- Minced garlic, 3 cloves
- Spiralized zucchini, 4
- Sliced mushrooms, 8 oz.
- Minced shallot, 2 tbsp.
- Cubed pancetta, 6 oz.
- EVOO, 4 tbsp. – divided

What to Do

1. Add two tablespoons of oil into a large skillet and let it heat up until it shimmers. Add in the pancetta and cook it until it has browned up. This will take about five minutes. With a slotted spoon, remove the pancetta and set it to the side.

2. Add in the rest of the oil and cook the mushrooms and shallot. Stir occasionally until they have browned up. This will take about five minutes. Mix in the zucchini and cook for three minutes more. The zucchini should become tender. Add in the garlic and cook until the garlic becomes fragrant. Make sure you stir constantly. Mix the pancetta back in and cook for another 30 seconds to warm the pancetta back up.

3. As the veggies are cooking, add the pepper, parmesan, cream, butter, and cream cheese to a pot. Heat and stir until everything has melted together. Whisk everything until they are heated through, about five minutes.

4. Divide the veggies between four containers, placing them to one side. Divide the sauce in the same containers, placing it on the other side. When ready to eat, mix the sauce and veggies together.

5. This will keep for four days in the refrigerator and six months in the freezer. Let it thaw overnight in the fridge. Place everything in a pot and heat everything together until warm. You may need to add in some cream to adjust the consistency.

Arroz Con Pollo

This recipe makes 4 servings and contains 513 calories; 35 g fat; 31 g protein; 13 g net carbs per serving

What You Need

- Sour cream, .5 c
- Shredded Monterey Jack, 1 c
- Uncooked cauliflower rice, 2 c
- Cayenne
- Salt, .5 tsp.
- Garlic powder, 1 tsp.
- Cumin, 1 tsp.
- Oregano, 1 tsp.
- Chili powder, 1 tbsp.
- Crushed tomatoes, 14 oz.
- Sliced mushrooms, 8 oz.
- Chopped onion
- Chopped boneless skinless chicken thighs, 1 lb.
- Avocado oil, .25 c

What to Do

1. Add the oil to a large skillet and heat it up until it shimmers.

2. Add in the chicken and cook them, stirring occasionally, until it has browned. This will take about five minutes. With a slotted spoon, take the chicken out and set it to the side.

3. Mix in the mushrooms and onion. Stir occasionally, until the veggies have browned up. This will take about five minutes.

4. Place the chicken back in the skillet, along with any juices that may have collected.

5. Mix in the cayenne, salt, garlic powder, cumin, oregano, chili powder, and the can of tomatoes with their juices. Stir everything together and allow it to come to a simmer.

6. Mix in the cauliflower and cook for five minutes, stirring occasionally.

7. Mix in the cheese, stirring until the cheese is melted and incorporated.

8. Divide the mixture between four containers. Serve with a garnish of sour cream.

9. This will keep for five days in the fridge or for six months in the freezer. Allow it to thaw in the refrigerator overnight and then microwave it for a few minutes.

Chopped Chicken Salad

This recipe makes 4 servings and contains 499 calories; 40 g fat; 22 g protein; 12 g net carbs per serving

What You Need

- Red pepper flakes
- Pepper
- Salt, .5 tsp.
- Minced shallot, 1 tbsp.
- Apple cider vinegar, 3 tbsp.
- EVOO, .5 c
- Dijon, 2 tbsp.
- Quartered cherry tomatoes, 8
- Chopped and drained artichoke hearts, 14 oz. can
- Chopped red bell pepper
- Sliced black olives, .5 c
- Chopped hard-boil eggs, 2
- Chopped meat from a rotisserie chicken, 1 lb.

What to Do

1. Mix together the cherry tomatoes, artichoke hearts, bell pepper, olives, eggs, and chicken in a large bowl.

2. Mix together the red pepper flakes, pepper, salt, shallot, vinegar, oil, and mustard.

3. Place the chicken salad equally into four storage containers. Divide the vinaigrette between four single-serving dressing containers. Toss the salad in the dressing to serve.

4. This won't freeze, but it will keep for a week in the refrigerator.

Simple Salmon Salad

This recipe makes 4 servings and contains 446 calories; 31 g fat; 34 g protein; 9 g net carbs per serving

What You Need

- Pepper
- Dried dill, 1 tsp.
- Zest and juice of a lemon
- Dijon, 1 tsp.
- EVOO, 3 tbsp.
- Mayonnaise, .5 c
- Chopped dill pickles, 3
- Chopped scallions, 3
- Flaked salmon, 8 oz. can

What to Do

1. Mix together the pickles, scallions, and salmon.

2. Beat together the pepper, dill, lemon zest and juice, mustard, oil, and mayonnaise.

3. Mix the salmon and the dressing together.

4. Divide the mixture between four storage containers.

5. This won't freeze, but you can keep it stored for five days in the refrigerator.

Gyro Salad with Tzatziki

This recipe makes 3 servings and contains 501 calories; 31 g fat; 47 g protein; 10 g net carbs per serving

What You Need

- Pepper, .5 tsp.
- Salt, .5 tsp.
- Chopped dill, 1 tsp.
- Chopped mint, 2 tsp.
- Ripe avocado
- Thyme, .5 tsp.
- Oregano, .5 tsp.
- Juice of a lemon – divided
- Low-sodium chicken broth, .25 c
- Grated cucumber, 1 medium
- Chopped onion, .5
- Olive oil, 1 tbsp.
- Ground lamb meat, 1 lb.
- Chopped romaine, 6 c

What to Do

1. Heat the oil in a large skillet. Once the oil has become hot, add in the lamb and cook for three minutes.

2. Mix in the onion. Cook until the onion has become soft.

3. Mix in the thyme, oregano, lemon juice, and chicken broth. Season with pepper and salt. Turn the heat up and allow it to simmer for five minutes.

4. Spread the grated cucumber out on a cheesecloth and squeeze as much liquid off of the cucumber as you can.

5. For the sauce, add the dill, mint, lemon juice, avocado, and cucumber to a food processor. Mix everything together until it becomes smooth.

6. Place the lettuce in three storage containers. Divide the lamb mixture between the same containers, making sure it stays to one side. Divide that sauce between three single-serving dressing containers. When you are ready to eat, pour the sauce over the meat and lettuce and toss together.

7. This should not be frozen unless you are storing the lamb mixture by itself. The lamb mixture will last five days in the refrigerator, and it can be frozen by itself for up to six months. The tzatziki sauce will last for a week in the refrigerator.

Pepperoni Pizza

This recipe makes 6 servings and contains 563 calories; 44 g fat; 33 g protein; 5 g net carbs per serving

What You Need

- Pepper, .25 tsp.
- Salt, .5 tsp.
- Italian seasoning, 2 tsp.
- Chopped basil, 3 tbsp.
- Pepperoni slices, 2 oz. – divided
- Shredded mozzarella, .5 c – divided
- Low-carb tomato sauce, .66 c – divided
- EVOO, 3 tbsp.
- Psyllium husk powder, .25 c
- Grated parmesan, 8 tbsp.
- Eggs, 6

What to Do

1. Add the Italian seasoning, psyllium powder, parmesan, and eggs in a blender.

2. Blend the mixture together until smooth, and then let it rest for five minutes.

3. Add a tablespoon of oil to a skillet.

4. Add in a third of the batter to the skillet. Cook the batter on both sides to create the crust. Do this twice more to use up the batter.

5. Place the crusts on a baking sheet and divide the tomato sauce over each crust.

6. Evenly divide the mozzarella and pepperoni on the crusts. Slide this under a broiler and cook until the cheese has melted and turned brown.

7. Sprinkle the top with some pepper, salt, and basil.

8. Allow the pizzas to cool off. Slice them each in half and place a half of a pizza into a storage container.

9. This will keep for five days in the refrigerator. This does not freeze well. To reheat, warm in the oven at 350 for ten minutes.

Double the Meat Stromboli

This recipe makes 6 servings and contains 533 calories; 38 g fat; 33 g protein; 7 g net carbs per serving

What You Need

- Pepper, .5 tsp.
- Salt, .5 tsp.
- Italian seasoning, 2 tsp.
- Coconut flour, .5 c
- Almond flour, .5 c
- Melted butter, 2 tbsp.
- Sliced cheddar, 1 c
- Sliced pepperoni, 4 oz.
- Sliced ham, 1 c
- Eggs, 2
- Shredded mozzarella, 2.5 c
- Salad greens, 12 c

What to Do

1. Start by placing your oven to 400.

2. Place parchment on a baking sheet.

3. Add the mozzarella to a microwave-safe bowl. Heat in 30-second increments until the cheese has melted, stirring each time until it becomes smooth.

4. Mix together the Italian seasoning, coconut flour, and almond flour.

5. Add in the melted cheese with the pepper and salt. Mix until everything has come together.

6. Stir in the eggs until the batter turns into dough.

7. Place this on the baking sheet. Lay another piece of parchment over top and use a rolling pin to roll the dough out into an oval shape.

8. Slice diagonal lines along the edges. Make sure that the middle four inches are not cut.

9. Layer the cheese, ham, and pepperoni in the middle of the dough. Fold the dough strips up over the toppings.

10. Brush the dough with some melted butter.

11. Slide the Stromboli into the oven and let it bake for 15-20 minutes or until it turns brown.

12. Slice the Stromboli into six equal sections.

13. Place a section into six containers. When you are ready to eat, serve with two cups of fresh salad greens.

14. I do not suggest freezing the Stromboli. It will keep in the fridge for five days.

Avocado Egg Salad

This recipe makes 6 servings and contains 348 calories; 28 g fat; 15 g protein; 4 g net carbs per serving

What You Need

- Pepper
- Salt
- Chopped red bell pepper, .5 pepper
- Chopped onion, .25
- Sliced avocados, 2
- Chopped hard-boiled eggs, 12

What to Do

1. Add the pepper, salt, bell pepper, onion, avocados, and eggs to a large bowl. Gently mix everything together until it is well-combined.

2. Divide the mixture between six storage containers.

3. This doesn't freeze well, but it will keep for five days in the refrigerator.

Herbed Turkey

This recipe makes 14 servings and contains 910 calories; 33 g fat; 47 g protein; 142 g net carbs per serving

What You Need

- Pepper, 1 tbsp.
- Salt, 1 tbsp.
- Whole garlic, 6 cloves
- Celery, 6 stalks
- Lemon, .5
- Large onion
- Thawed turkey, 15 lb.
- Coconut oil, 3 tbsp.
- Herbed Butter:
- Chopped parsley, .25 c
- Rosemary, 1 tbsp.
- Minced garlic, 4 cloves
- Butter, .5 c

What to Do

1. Place the herbed butter ingredients in a bowl and mix everything together. Set to the side but do not refrigerate.

2. Set your oven to 325.

3. Clean out the turkey cavities and rinse it with cold water until it runs clear. Pat the turkey dry.

4. Set the turkey in a large roasting pan that has been fitted with a roasting rack.

5. Place the celery, onion, garlic, and lemon wedges inside of the turkey.

6. Rub the turkey with the herbed butter and then drizzle the coconut oil over the top of the turkey.

7. Slide the turkey in the oven.

8. The turkey needs to cook for at least 20 minutes per pound. This will be around five hours. Check the temperature during the last few hours because it could get done early, and you don't want the turkey to dry out. It needs to reach 165.

9. Remove the cooked turkey and allow it to rest for at least ten minutes before you carve.

10. If you are meal prepping, separate the carved meat equally between 14 storage containers.

11. This can be frozen for up to six months. When you reheat, you can use some more herbed butter to add moisture and flavor.

Tilapia with Avocado Salad

This recipe makes 8 servings and contains 382 calories; 23 g fat; 37 g protein; 6 g net carbs per serving

What You Need

- Halved cherry tomatoes, 1 c
- Diced avocado, 1 c
- Oregano, 1 tsp.
- Lemon zest, 2 tbsp.
- Lemon juice, 4 tbsp.
- Pepper, .5 tsp.
- Salt, .5 tsp.
- Minced garlic, 2 cloves
- Greek yogurt, 2 tbsp.
- Coconut oil, 5 tbsp.
- Tilapia fillets, 8 6-oz. fillets

What to Do

1. Mix together the pepper, salt, garlic, yogurt, lemon zest, and lemon juice. Stir in the coconut oil until everything comes together.

2. Place the tilapia in a bowl or a bag and cover with the yogurt mixture. Make sure that the fish is very well-coated.

3. Allow the fish to sit in the fridge for 20 minutes or overnight.

4. Set your oven to 400.

5. Lay the fish in a baking dish and slide it into the oven.

6. Bake the fish for 10-12 minutes. The fillets should easily flake with a fork.

7. Mix together a tablespoon of coconut oil with the tomatoes and avocados.

8. Using eight containers, place a tilapia fillet and a half of a cup of the salad.

9. This will keep for five days in the refrigerator. I do not suggest freezing. Reheat the fish by itself in the microwave for a couple of minutes.

Fish Tacos

This recipe makes 4 servings and contains 301 calories; 21 g fat; 25 g protein; 2 g net carbs per serving

What You Need

- Large lettuce leaves, 4
- Minced chipotle peppers in adobo, 2
- Sliced jalapeno
- Chopped onion
- Olive oil, 2 tbsp.
- Butter, 2 tbsp.
- Mayonnaise, 2 tbsp.
- Coconut oil, 2 tbsp.
- Crushed garlic, 2 cloves
- Tilapia, 1 lb.

What to Do

1. Add two tablespoons of coconut oil to a skillet.

2. Once hot, add the onions and let them cook for about five minutes, or until they become translucent.

3. Turn the heat down and then mix in the garlic and jalapeno. Cook this for another two minutes, stirring occasionally. A word of advice, don't let your face be directly over the pan when you add the jalapeno. The fumes from the pepper will burn your eyes and throat.

4. Mince up the chipotle and mix them into the other vegetables.

5. Place the fish fillets in the skillet with the butter and mayonnaise.

6. Mix everything together and let it all cook together for eight minutes, or until the fish is cooked through.

7. To make your tacos, divide the fish mixture between the lettuce leaves.

8. For meal prep, divide the fish mixture between four containers. When ready to eat, heat the fish and wrap it in a lettuce leaf.

9. This will keep for five days in the refrigerator. Do not freeze this dish.

Herbed Salmon

This recipe makes 4 servings and contains 211 calories; 12 g fat; 22 g protein; 1 g net carbs per serving

What You Need

- Sliced lemon, 2
- Onion powder, .5 tsp.
- Pepper, .5 tsp.
- Salt, .5 tsp.
- Olive oil, 2 tbsp.
- Whole garlic, 4 cloves
- Rosemary, 4 springs
- Chopped thyme, 1 tbsp.
- Chopped basil, 1 tbsp.
- Chopped parsley, 1 tbsp.
- Boneless salmon, 4 6-oz. fillets

What to Do

1. Start by placing your oven to 400.

2. Mix together the onion powder, pepper, salt, olive oil, thyme, basil, and parsley. Make sure it is very well-combined.

3. Place foil on a baking sheet and spray with cooking spray. Lay the salmon fillets on the baking sheet.

4. Rub the herbed mixture into the fish and top the salmon with lemon slices, a whole garlic clove, and a sprig of rosemary.

5. Slide this into the oven for 10-13 minutes. The salmon should flake easily with a fork.

6. For meal prep, place a salmon fillet in a storage container.

7. This should not be frozen, but it will keep in the fridge for five days.

Coconut Shrimp Soup

This recipe makes 4 servings and contains 289 calories; 26 g fat; 13 g protein; 3 g net carbs per serving

What You Need

- Pepper, .5 tsp.
- Salt, .5 tsp.
- Chopped cilantro, 2 tbsp.
- Grated ginger, 1 tsp.
- Basil, 1 tbsp.
- Fish sauce, 1 tbsp.
- Fish stock, 3 c
- Minced garlic, 4 cloves
- Chopped onion
- Melted coconut oil, 1 tbsp.
- Thai coconut milk, 14 oz. can
- Lime juice, 1 tbsp.
- Cleaned shrimp, 1 lb.

What to Do

1. Add the coconut oil to a large pot. Add in the garlic and onion. Cook for about six minutes, or until they have softened. Stir occasionally and don't let the garlic burn.

2. Add in the shrimp, cook, stirring occasionally until the shrimp turn pink.

3. Gently mix in all of the other ingredients and bring everything to a boil.

4. Once it has started to boil, lower the heat, and let it cook for 15 minutes at a simmer. Stir occasionally. Taste and adjust any of the seasonings that you need to.

5. Divide soup between four containers.

6. This can be kept for five months in the refrigerator. You can also store it in the freezer for six months. Let the soup thaw out in the fridge and reheat it in a pot until warmed through.

Crab Cakes

This recipe makes 4 servings and contains 303 calories; 18 g fat; 16 g protein; 3 g net carbs per serving

What You Need

- Chopped parsley, 1 tbsp.
- Paprika, .25 tsp.
- Garlic powder, .25 tsp.
- Onion powder, .25 tsp.
- Pepper, .5 tsp.
- Salt, .5 tsp.
- Mayonnaise, .25 c
- Dijon, 1 tsp.
- Butter, 4 tbsp.
- Coconut flour, 1 c
- Lump crab meat, 1.5 lb.

What You Need

1. Mix together the parsley, paprika, garlic powder, onion powder, pepper, salt, Dijon, and mayonnaise together.

2. Mix in the crab meat and make sure that everything is well combined and the crab is completely coated.

3. Slowly mix in the flour and stir everything together with your hands. Form the mixture into four patties.

4. Add the butter to a skillet, and once heated, place the crab cake in the pan and cook for four to six minutes on each side. Repeat this until all of the patties are cooked.

5. Place a crab cake into individual containers.

6. This cannot be frozen. This can be kept refrigerated for five days.

Specialty, Dessert, and Snacks

Almond Joy Fat Bomb

This recipe makes 12 servings and contains 188 calories; 21 g fat; <1 g protein; 2 g net carbs per serving

What You Need

- Liquid stevia
- Coconut oil, 1 c
- Unsweetened baking chocolate, 2 oz.
- Almond butter, 1 c

What to Do

1. Mix all of the ingredients together in a pot. Cook and stir the mixture until everything has melted and mixed together. Taste and add extra stevia if you need to.

2. Pour this mixture into mini muffin tins, ice cube trays, or candy molds.

3. Chill the fat bombs for at least an hour. Remove the fat bombs from their molds and keep them in a storage container.

4. These will last for five days in the refrigerator or for six months in the freezer.

Strawberry Ice Pops

This recipe makes 4 servings and contains 272 calories; 27 g fat; 3 g protein; 6 g net carbs per serving

What You Need

- Liquid stevia, .5 tsp.
- Full-fat coconut milk, 13.6 oz. can
- Halved strawberries, 1 c

What to Do

1. Combine all of the ingredients together in a food processor or blender. Mix until the mixture becomes smooth.

2. Pour the mixture into ice pop molds and allow them to freeze overnight before you serve them.

3. This will keep in the freezer for six months.

Coconut Mousse

This recipe makes 6 servings and contains 396 calories; 41 g fat; 5 g protein; 6 g net carbs per serving

What You Need

- Vanilla, .5 tsp.
- Liquid stevia, 1 tsp.
- Espresso powder, 1 tsp.
- Melted and cooled unsweetened baking chocolate, 2 oz.
- Coconut milk, 2 13.6-oz. cans – use only the cream but reserve some of the milk if needed to reach your desired consistency

What to Do

1. Whisk all of the ingredients together until they are well combined. Use some of the coconut water if you need to thin out the mousse a little bit.

2. Divide the mouse between six containers.

3. This can keep for five days in the refrigerator. You can also freeze the mixture and slice it into six squares to make fudge.

Stuffed Mushrooms

This recipe makes 8 servings and contains 162 calories; 13 g fat; 9 g protein; 4 g net carbs per serving

What You Need

- Stemmed button mushrooms, 1 lb.
- Parmesan, .5 c
- Minced shallot, 1 tbsp.
- Garlic powder, 1 tsp.
- Tabasco, 2 dashes
- Dijon, 1 tsp.
- Chopped frozen spinach, 4 oz. – thawed and wrung dry
- Room temperature cream cheese, 8 oz.

What to Do

1. Start by placing your oven to 425.

2. Mix together the parmesan, shallot, garlic powder, Tabasco, mustard, spinach, and cream cheese.

3. Lay the mushrooms in a baking sheet with the cap-side down.

4. Spoon a generous amount of the filling into each of the mushroom caps.

5. Allow this to bake for 25 minutes. Allow the mushrooms to cool off.

6. Divide the mushrooms into eight storage containers.

7. These won't freeze, but they keep in the refrigerator for five days. You can reheat in the microwave for a couple of minutes or for 25 minutes in an oven at 350.

Onion Dip with Crudités

This recipe makes 6 servings and contains 211 calories; 18 g fat; 4 g protein; 8 g net carbs per serving

What You Need

- Sliced bell peppers, 2
- Dijon, 1 tsp.
- Mayonnaise, .25 c
- Room temperature cream cheese, 8 oz.
- Salt, .5 tsp.
- Thyme, 1 tsp.
- Thinly sliced onions, 2
- Avocado oil, .25 c

What to Do

1. Add the oil to a skillet and heat until the oil begins to shimmer.

2. Turn the heat down, and then add in the salt, thyme, and onions.

3. Cook the onions, stirring occasionally, until they have caramelized. This will take 20-30 minutes. Allow the onions to cool off.

4. Add the mustard, mayonnaise, cream cheese, and onions to a bowl and mix everything together. Make sure that everything is evenly distributed.

5. Using six storage containers, add a quarter cup of dip. In six more storage containers, divide out the pepper strips. Even the pepper strips dipped into the onion dip.

6. The dip won't freeze, but it will all last about three days in the refrigerator.

Jalapeno Poppers

This recipe makes 8 servings and contains 240 calories; 20 g fat; 12 g protein; 3 g net carbs per serving

What You Need

- Crumbled cooked bacon, 8 slices
- Jalapeno peppers cut lengthwise with the ribs and seeds removed, 16
- Shredded pepper jack cheese, .5 c
- Room temperature cream cheese, 6 oz.

What to Do

1. Start by placing your oven to 350.

2. Mix together the pepper jack cheese and the cream cheese until smooth.

3. Spoon this into the jalapeno halves and then lay them, with the cheese up, on a baking sheet. Sprinkle the bacon over the top of the cheese.

4. Bake the jalapeno poppers for 25 minutes, or until the cheese has melted and is bubbly.

5. Place four cooled poppers in eight storage containers.

6. These will keep in the fridge for five days. They don't freeze well. You can heat them up for two minutes in the microwave or 15-20 minutes at 350 in the oven.

Deviled Eggs

This recipe makes 6 servings and contains 72 calories; 6 g fat; 3 g protein; 3 g net carbs per serving

What You Need

- Salt, .5 tsp.
- Minced garlic, 1 clove
- Cayenne
- Minced scallions, 2
- Minced dill pickle
- Dijon, 1 tsp.
- Mayonnaise, .5 c
- Halved hard-boiled eggs, 6

What to Do

1. Remove the yolks from the whites and place them in a bowl. Lay the whites on a plate with the cut side up.

2. Mix together the salt, garlic, cayenne, scallions, pickle, mustard, mayonnaise, and yolks. Use a fork so that you can mash up the yolks as you go. Mix until they are well combined.

3. Place the yolk mixture into the egg whites either with a spoon or a piping bag.

4. Place two deviled eggs into six storage containers.

5. These will last for five days in the refrigerator.

Green Bean Casserole

This recipe makes 4 servings and contains 366 calories; 31 g fat; 15 g protein; 12 g net carbs per serving

What You Need

- Shredded cheddar, .5 c
- Caramelized onions, .5 c
- Cream of mushroom soup, 10.5 oz. can
- Cooked green beans, 3 c

What to Do

1. Start by placing your oven to 350.

2. Mix together all of the ingredients in a large bowl.

3. Spread the green bean mixture into the bottom of a 9" x 13" casserole dish. Bake the casserole for 15 minutes, or until it is hot and bubbly.

4. Allow the casserole to cool before you place it into storage containers.

5. Add a cup of the casserole to four storage containers.

6. This will keep in the refrigerator for five days. It doesn't freeze well. To heat it, bake it for 15 minutes at 350, or microwave it for a couple of minutes.

Roasted Brussels Sprouts

This recipe makes 4 servings and contains 347 calories; 26 g fat; 16 g protein; 10 g net carbs per serving

What You Need

- Pepper
- Salt, .5 tsp.
- Chopped bacon, 4 oz.
- Halved Brussels sprouts, 1.5 lbs.
- Avocado oil, .25 c

What to Do

1. Start by placing your oven to 400.

2. Toss together the pepper, salt, bacon, sprouts, and oil together so that the sprouts are well coated.

3. Lay the sprouts out on a baking sheet and bake them for 20 minutes. Flip the sprouts over halfway through the cooking time. You want them to brown up on both sides.

4. Once cooled, divide between four storage containers.

5. These will keep for five days in the refrigerator. You can freeze them, but the texture will become mushy once you reheat.

Mashed Cauliflower

This recipe makes 4 servings and contains 143 calories; 14 g fat; 3 g protein; 3 g net carbs per serving

What You Need

- Pepper
- Salt, .5 tsp.
- Heavy cream, .25 c
- Melted butter, .25 c
- Head of cauliflower

What to Do

1. Break apart the head of cauliflower into florets and place them in a pot of water and cover with water. Bring this to a boil.

2. Allow the cauliflower to boil for ten minutes, or until the cauliflower is soft.

3. Drain off the water. Place the cauliflower in a bowl and mash with a potato masher. Mix in the pepper, salt, cream, and butter. Mix until everything is incorporated and smooth.

4. Divide the mashed cauliflower between four containers.

5. You can keep in the refrigerator for five days or freeze it up to six months. Thaw it in the refrigerator overnight and then microwave for a couple of minutes to heat through. You can also heat it up on the stovetop. You may want to add a bit of cream to adjust the consistency.

Chopped Caprese Salad

This recipe makes 4 servings and contains 373 calories; 28 g fat; 25 g protein; 6 g net carbs per serving

What You Need

- Pepper
- Salt, .5 tsp.
- EVOO, .25 c
- Chopped mozzarella, 12 oz.
- Chopped basil leaves, 1 bunch
- Chopped heirloom tomatoes, 3 large

What to Do

1. Toss all of the ingredients together in a large bowl. Divide the salad between four containers.

2. Do not freeze this. It will keep, refrigerated, for three days.

Coleslaw

This recipe makes 4 servings and contains 103 calories; 7 g fat; 2 g protein; 7 g net carbs per serving

What You Need

- Salt, .5 tsp.
- Grated ginger, 1 tsp.
- Minced garlic clove
- Sesame seeds, 1 tbsp.
- Chinese hot mustard, .5 tsp.
- Sriracha, .5 tsp.
- Juice of a lime
- Avocado oil, .5 c
- Apple cider vinegar, .25 c
- Chopped cilantro, 1 bunch
- Chopped scallions, 6
- Shredded cabbage, 4 c

What to Do

1. Toss together the cilantro, scallions, and cabbage.

2. Whisk together the salt, ginger, garlic, sesame seeds, mustard, sriracha, lime juice, oil, and vinegar.

3. Add a cup of the cabbage mixture to four storage containers. Using four single-serving dressing containers, add three tablespoons of the dressing. When you are ready to serve, toss the cabbage in the dressing.

4. Do not freeze this. The dressing will keep for a week in the fridge, and the slaw will last five days.

Fat Bomb Vanilla Smoothie

This recipe makes 4 servings and contains 551 calories; 48 g fat; 28 g protein; 6 g net carbs per serving

What You Need

- Vanilla, 1 tsp.
- Powdered erythritol, 2 tbsp.
- Coconut oil, 3 tbsp.
- Ice cubes, 8
- Vanilla almond milk, .5 c
- Whipped cream, .5 c
- Heavy cream, 1 c
- Vanilla protein powder, 2 scoops

What to Do

1. Add all of the ingredients to your blender except for the whipped cream.

2. Blend the ingredients together for a minute, or until they become smooth.

3. Pour the mixture into four glasses and top with the whipped cream.

4. If you are meal prepping, pour the smoothie mixture into cupcake tins. Freeze the mixture and pop a few out when you want a smoothie. Blend them together and enjoy.

Homemade Nutella

This recipe makes 24 servings and contains 173 calories; 33 g fat; 3 g protein; 2 g net carbs per serving

What You Need

- Salt, .25 tsp.
- Stevia, .5 c
- Vanilla, 1 tsp.
- Unsweetened coconut milk, .5 c
- Heavy cream, .5 c
- Coconut oil, 4 tbsp.
- Unsweetened cacao powder, .5 c
- Hazelnuts, 4 c

What to Do

1. Start by placing your oven to 325.

2. Place the hazelnuts on a cookie sheet and slide them in the oven. Roast the nuts for 10-15 minutes or until they have browned up.

3. Place the hazelnuts on a wet towel and rub them until the dark skin has come off.

4. Add the hazelnuts and all of the other ingredients to a blender and mix until it forms a smooth mixture.

5. Keep this stored in a mason jar.

6. Keep this in the refrigerator and will likely last a month if it doesn't get eaten faster. Spread two tablespoons on some berries, or add to a smoothie.

Peanut Butter Cookies

This recipe makes 15 servings and contains 107 calories; 10 g fat; 5 g protein; 2 g net carbs per serving

What You Need

- Salt
- Erythritol, .5 c
- Egg
- Peanut butter, 1 c

What to Do

1. Start by setting your oven to 350.

2. Place parchment paper on a baking sheet.

3. Stir together all of the ingredients until they are well combined.

4. Form 15 1-inch balls of cookie dough and place them on the baking sheet.

5. Press them down a bit with a fork and slide them into the oven.

6. Let the cookies bake for 10-15 minutes, or until the edges have browned up. If you like crispy cookies, cook for a bit longer. If you like soft cookies, don't cook them quite as long.

7. These will keep at room temp for a week. You can also freeze them for up to six months. Allow them to come to room temperature before eating.

Cloud Bread

This recipe makes 10 servings and contains 50 calories; 6 g fat; 3 g protein; 0 g net carbs per serving

What You Need

- Softened cream cheese, 3 oz.
- Cream of tartar, .25 tsp.
- Separated eggs, 3

What to Do

1. Start by placing your oven to 300.

2. Place parchment on a baking sheet.

3. Separate the eggs, placing the yolks and whites in separate bowls.

4. Add the cream of tartar to the egg whites and whip until they are fluffy and shiny.

5. Beat the cream cheese into the yolks until well mixed. Carefully fold the fluffy whites into the yolks.

6. Spoon out ten circles of the batter onto the baking sheet. Make sure that you keep them two inches apart so that they don't run into each other.

7. Slide these into the oven and bake them for 30 minutes or until they are browned and firm.

8. Keep these stored in the refrigerator. Do not freeze them. This will cause the bread to fall.

Parfait

This recipe makes 4 servings and contains 353 calories; 23 g fat; 22 g protein; 5 g net carbs per serving

What You Need

- Toasted flaxseeds, 1 c
- Sliced bananas, 4 medium
- Blueberries, 2 c
- Sliced strawberries, 2 c
- Full-fat yogurt, 4 c
- Desiccated coconut, 1 c
- Chopped macadamia nuts, 1 c
- Chopped toasted walnuts, 1.5 c

What to Do

1. With four mason jars, add a half cup of yogurt into the bottom of each.

2. Layer the flaxseeds, bananas, blueberries, strawberries, coconut, macadamia nuts, and walnuts into each of the jars.

3. Top each with another half cup of yogurt.

4. Keep these stored in the refrigerator for three days.

Peanut Butter Chocolate Chip Cookies

This recipe makes 16 servings and contains 215 calories; 13 g fat; 6 g protein; 2 g net carbs per serving

What You Need

- Sea salt
- Vanilla, 1 tsp.
- Cinnamon, 1 tbsp.
- Baking powder, 1 tsp.
- Eggs, 2
- Truvia, .75 c
- Butter, .5 c
- Unsweetened chocolate chips, 1.5 c
- Peanut butter, 1 c
- Unsweetened coconut milk, 2 tbsp.
- Coconut flour, 3 c

What to Do

1. Start by setting your oven to 350.

2. Mix together the salt, coconut, vanilla, cinnamon, egg, butter, chocolate chips, peanut butter, milk, and flour. Make sure that everything is mixed together.

3. Roll the dough into 16 1.5-inch balls.

4. Place the dough on the cookie sheet and slide into the oven. Allow the cookies to bake for 15 minutes. You can adjust the cooking time depending on how soft or crispy you want your cookies.

5. Take the cookies out of the oven and allow them to cool.

6. Keep the cookies in a lidded bowl or a Ziploc bag at room temperature. They will last a week.

Berry Cheesecake

This recipe makes 6 servings and contains 431 calories; 40 g fat; 13 g protein; 3 g net carbs per serving

What You Need

Crust:

- Vanilla, 1 tsp.
- Stevia, 3 tbsp.
- Melted coconut oil, .33 c
- Coconut flour, 2 c

Filling:

- Salt, .5 tsp.
- Vanilla, 1 tsp.
- Lemon juice, 1 tbsp.
- Powdered erythritol, 1.25 c
- Cream cheese, 4 8-oz. pack
- Eggs, 3
- Topping:
- Powdered erythritol
- Mixed berries, 1-2 c

What to Do

1. Start by placing your oven to 350.

2. Mix together the vanilla, stevia, butter, and coconut flours. Grease a springform pan and press the crust into the pan.

3. Bake the crust for ten minutes. Allow the crust to cool for at least ten minutes before putting anything in it.

4. Beat the cream cheese with an electric mixture. Add in the eggs, beating until completely combined.

5. Beat in the salt, vanilla, lemon juice, and powdered erythritol. Mix until completely combined.

6. Pour the filling into the pan and smooth the top out.

7. Place the cheesecake in the oven and bake it for 50 minutes.

8. Carefully remove the cheesecake and cool for 30 minutes. Remove the cake from the pan.

9. Mix the erythritol and berries together and pour over top of the cheesecake.

10. Keep the cake refrigerated. It will last a week.

Chocolate Cake

This recipe makes 6 servings and contains 347 calories; 32 g fat; 9 g protein; 2 g net carbs per serving

What You Need

- Erythritol, 1 c
- Baking powder, 1 tsp.
- Baking soda, 1 tsp.
- Unsweetened coconut milk, .5 c
- Eggs, 6
- Softened butter, .75 c
- Unsweetened cocoa powder, .5 c
- Coconut flour, 3.5 c
- Frosting:
- Salt
- Vanilla, 1 tsp.
- Powdered erythritol, .66 c
- Softened butter, .33 c
- Melted unsweetened chocolate chips, .5 c
- Softened cream cheese, 2 8-oz. packs

What to Do

1. Start by placing your oven to 350.

2. Place parchment in a springform pan.

3. Mix together the erythritol, baking powder, baking soda, coconut milk, eggs, butter, cocoa powder, and coconut flour. Mix until it comes together.

4. Pour this into the springform pan and bake it for 25 minutes. A toothpick should come out clean.

5. Meanwhile, beat together the salt, vanilla, powdered erythritol, butter, and melted chocolate chips.

6. Take the cake out of the oven. Allow it to cool off for a few minutes, and then remove it from the pan. Once the cake is completely cooled, spread the frosting over it.

7. The cake will last a week in the refrigerator.

Lemon Bundt Cake

This recipe makes 8 servings and contains 391 calories; 23 g fat; 8 g protein; 5 g net carbs per serving

What You Need

- Salt, .5 tsp.
- Nutmeg, .25 tsp.
- Cinnamon, .5 tsp.
- Vanilla, .5 tsp.
- Baking powder, 1 tsp.
- Baking soda, 1 tsp.
- Raspberries, 2.5 c
- Powdered erythritol, 1 c
- Beaten eggs, 3
- Melted coconut oil, .5 c
- Lemon zest, 3 tsp.
- Coconut milk, 1 c
- Coconut flour, 3 c

What to Do

1. Start by placing your oven to 350.

2. Mix together the salt, nutmeg, cinnamon, vanilla, baking powder, baking soda, erythritol, eggs, coconut oil, lemon zest, coconut milk, and coconut flour. Stir until everything is well combined.

3. Carefully fold the raspberries in.

4. Spray a Bundt pan with cooking spray.

5. Pour the prepared batter into the Bundt pan.

6. Wrap the top of the pan with foil.

7. Slide the pan into the oven and bake it for 20 minutes. A toothpick should come out clean.

8. Allow the Bundt pan to cool off completely, and then carefully flip over onto a plate to remove.

9. This will keep for a week at room temperature.

Blueberry Pudding

This recipe makes 6 servings and contains 132 calories; 14 g fat; 4 g protein; 4 g net carbs per serving

What You Need

- Salt
- Vanilla, .25 tsp.
- Lemon juice, 1 tbsp.
- Coconut oil, 2 tbsp.
- Desiccated coconut, 1 c
- Chia seeds, .5 c
- Blueberries, 2 c
- Unsweetened coconut cream, .5 c
- Unsweetened coconut milk, 3 c

What to Do

1. Mix the coconut milk and coconut cream together.

2. Mix in the salt, vanilla, lemon juice, coconut, coconut oil, chia seeds, and blueberries until everything is well combined.

3. Divide the pudding between six containers and refrigerate for at least four hours before servings.

4. This will keep for five days in the refrigerator.

Berry Popsicles

This recipe makes 6 servings and contains 88 calories; 2 g fat; 4 g protein; 2 g net carbs per serving

What You Need

- Liquid stevia, 20-25 drops
- Heavy cream, .25 c
- Sour cream, .25 c
- Unsweetened coconut milk, 1 c
- Coconut oil, .25 c
- Blueberries, 1 c
- Strawberries, 1 c

What to Do

1. Add all of the ingredients to a blender and mix until smooth. You can adjust the sweetness as needed.

2. Pour the mixture through a mesh sieve into a measuring c. Push the mixture through to help clean out the seeds.

3. Pour this into popsicle molds and allow them to freeze at least two hours or until solid.

Chocolate Pudding

This recipe makes 6 servings and contains 198 calories; 17 g fat; 4 g protein; 2 g net carbs per serving

What You Need

- Stevia
- Salt
- Vanilla, .5 tsp.
- Cayenne, .5 tsp.
- Unsweetened coconut milk, 4 tbsp.
- Cinnamon, 4 tsp.
- Unsweetened cacao powder, .5 c
- Avocados, 4

What to Do

1. Place the avocados into a food processor and pulse until they are almost smooth.

2. Add in all of the rest of the ingredients and pulse until they are all mixed and smooth.

3. Pour the mixture into six mason jars. Refrigerate until they are chilled and serve.

4. They will keep in the fridge for three days.

Conclusion

Thanks for making it through to the end of *Keto Meal Prep 2021*. Let's hope it was informative and able to provide you with all of the tools you need to achieve your goals whatever they may be.

I hope you have found all the information you need to achieve your keto meal prep goals. You now understand the basics of a ketogenic diet and what it takes to be successful. You can use any of the meal prep plans I provided, or you can use the recipes to create a meal prep plan all on your own.

The important thing to remember is that following a ketogenic diet isn't some fad diet that will fade away with time. It is a lifestyle change that is going to improve your body. This diet's main purpose is to change your body's fuel source from fat to ketones by reducing your carb intake. After your body has reached ketosis, losing weight won't be as much of a pain.

You now know what it takes to live a healthy and satisfying life. Act now, and use the information found within these pages to make your life healthier and easier. There is no shortage of recipes, either. You will be amazed at how quickly your life and body can change when you start a ketogenic diet.

Finally, if you found this book useful in any way, a review is always appreciated!

www.ingramcontent.com/pod-product-compliance
Lightning Source LLC
Chambersburg PA
CBHW080419030426
42335CB00020B/2504